Breaking Free

A Guide to Recovering from Chronic Fatigue Syndrome and Long Covid Symptoms

Jan Rothney

**Breaking Free from Chronic Fatigue
and Long Covid Symptoms**
by Jan Rothney

© Jan Rothney

ISBN: 9781912092154

First published in 2022
by Arkbound Foundation (Publishers)

Arkbound is a social enterprise that aims to promote social inclusion, community development and artistic talent. It sponsors publications by disadvantaged authors and covers issues that engage wider social concerns. Arkbound fully embraces sustainability and environmental protection. It endeavours to use material that is renewable, recyclable or sourced from sustainable forest.

Arkbound, Rogart Street Campus
4 Rogart Street, Glasgow, G40 2AA
www.arkbound.com

Breaking Free

Jan Rothney

Acknowledgements

Thank you to so many people who have enabled me to get this far and be healthy! To my wonderful GP, Dr Steve Chevasse, for believing I could recover, and for contacting me at home when I was too weak to attend the surgery. And thank you Tracey Moore for being such a great nurse, reassurance and support.

My biggest thank you goes to my amazing girls, Amy and Kate, who had to manage on their own when I was upstairs recovering, and who regularly popped in to check on me. You have been my motivation, my greatest joy, and have been the only ones to be there throughout the whole bumpy journey. Telling me I need to listen to "The Hunter" by Dido and saying "we don't care if we live in a caravan as long as you are healthy", were game changers for me. I am so privileged to be your mum and so unbelievably proud of both of you.

A big thank you to the fabulous friends who kept me in the loop and visited, even when I was bedridden or too weak to go out: Barbara Hartley, Clarice Harwood, Bernadette Goan and my amazing cousin Gillian Leonard, who flew all the way from Ireland to see me. A massive thank you to my neighbour at that time, James Braddick, for endless shopping, phone calls and visits to check on me and the girls. To Barbara and Henry Hartley for doing the shopping, checking on the girls, and for doing the school run when I was bedridden.

During my relapse, I'd like to also thank the Oakley clan: Beth, Jim, Joe and Sam, who I am so fortunate to have in my life. Also, to Seb, for being so kind and caring when he visited.

Thank you to Neil Davidson for telling me to stop talking about it and start writing my book, and for putting me in touch with The Book Midwife, Mindy Gibbons-Klein and Alex Pink - media production expert extraordinaire. I never dreamt I would write my first draft in seven weeks on this writing course with Mindy. Thank you. I am so grateful to those who test read my first draft of certain chapters and gave me valuable feedback: Anna Rutherford, Alan Mead, Cat Paterson, Sarah Freeman, Ben Fisk, Sarah Flegg and Sophie Hartwell. Also, Barbara Hartley, Jill Stokes and Lyn Friend for incredible support with final corrections. Thank you also to Thom Stokes, who gave me lots of research into Vitamin D3 and its impact on the immune system, and for our fabulous nerdy chats.

Amanda Thomas, journalist, broadcaster, and writer was instrumental in getting the book published, as she kindly introduced my book to Arkbound Publishers. A massive thank you to Arkbound for accepting my book and taking me through the whole process. The team at Arkbound have been so supportive, especially Steve McNaught, Jamie Nixon and Elsie Elder. It means so much to me to be published and share the message of how to recover and stay robust.

The stunning illustrations in this book are by Jenna Green (www.jennagreenart.com), who has been incredibly helpful throughout the whole process. *Breaking Free from Chronic Fatigue and Long Covid Symptoms* would not be the same without her genius. Alex Pink (www.pinkphotovideo.com) has transformed my amateur scribbles into professional diagrams for you and has been thought-provoking throughout. Alex is also doing all the videos for the *Reset to Thrive* online programme. I want to thank Elly Donavan, publicist, for her invaluable help and for putting me in touch with Vicky Edwards and Duncan Barkes, media trainers. Also, to Tasmin Briers for the beautiful front cover.

A sincere thank you to my incredible, lovely husband, who has always encouraged me to do what is important for me, who loves me for who I am, warts and all, and who has given me the time and the space to write and supported me throughout my edits. I am unbelievably lucky to have met you and I never take for granted how lucky I am. You have no idea how much your gentle nature, your kindness to everyone, and your stability have kept me healthy and happy. You are my rock.

And a huge thank you to my wonderful clients who have been inspirational, stimulating, fun and a joy to work with and to those who contributed to the book. Finally, to any sufferer and their health practitioners, employers, or carers who read this book and find it useful for understanding and dealing with recovery. I have always wanted to share ideas on how to recover and you have enabled me to spread the word.

Introduction

*"Whether you think you can, or you think you can't -
you're right." - Henry Ford, 1922*

There is no magic in my work, just the incredible magic of the body itself. When I was diagnosed with Myalgic Encephalomyelitis (M.E.) in 2002, I lay in bed helpless and immobilised, housebound for months, after an onslaught of various viruses, injuries, lack of sleep and conflict. Thankfully, my background in health and social care meant that I knew why my body had shut itself down, and how to get it going again. That's precisely what I did, with the constant reassurance of my GP. If I recovered on my own, then the good news is that you can too! This book shares everything I used to recover.

When I had a relapse in 2005, I was devastated. Then, instead of seeing my GP, I was referred to a new chronic fatigue syndrome (CFS) team. They told me I would *not* recover; I would never be the person I was, and that I would have to learn to accept and 'manage' the illness. It made me feel powerless and incapable of recovery. Thankfully, I found someone who reminded me I *can* recover, and I did. After heading for a third relapse a few years later, I realised I had to change my life and went on to have permanent health and fitness, as many others do. Even today, so many GPs and specialists do not understand post viral fatigue syndrome (PVFS), Fibromyalgia (FM), and now Long Covid.

It has been my ambition to write a book since retiring from my practice in 2019 because it is wrong, and harmful, to tell people they can't recover. I want to let people know they can recover, be completely healthy again, and *stay* healthy. I have worked with many people in my clinic, who have made some incredible recoveries; people who came to me blindfolded, due to light sensitivity, in pain or who were unable to go out, without the aid of a wheelchair.

If they can, *you* can. Consider the case of Mick as the first one to inspire you:-

> *Mick, a young mountain bike champion, was terrified when I first worked with him. He wore a blindfold, because of light sensitivity, and had a timer to limit our first session to 10 minutes because any activity exhausted him.*
>
> *Thankfully, Mick agreed to trust me to proceed without using a timer and we did an hour session before taking a break. For the first time in a year, he went outside and walked down his driveway. To him, it seemed like a miracle, but it was the body doing exactly what the body is meant to do, when it knows it is safe. He has now been back in full-time employment for many years and lives a normal life.*

If this excites you, and you want to be like him and thousands of others who recover, then read on. And if, like Mick, you notice that you put limits on activities, anticipate disaster and are convinced you will become more ill if you do anything, you will benefit hugely from the chapters on "How to Recover".

It doesn't matter whether you have had the condition for six months or 20 years; the people who recover are the ones who discover that there is a way, which they hadn't known before, and are eager to learn it.

> *One lady, called Margaret, had been ill for over 20 years: she led a minimal life, had to use a wheelchair when moving around, and was almost completely bed bound.*
>
> *For our first session, she was excited and so determined to do well that she refused the wheelchair and, using a walking stick, walked a full five metres. I knew, as soon as I saw her*

determination, that this woman had a high chance of doing well, no matter how long she had been ill.

The body will naturally heal when you do what it takes to recover. We will revisit Margaret's story to find out what she did that was so effective for recovery.

Many people get stuck after a virus, a trauma or, today, Covid-19. If this is you, it will become clear how to get better and regain your health.

It is my mission to show you that you can recover like Margaret, Mick and others. I want to give you and any professionals involved with the illness all the components needed to recover and to stay healthy and robust.

Part One is how I recovered on my own the first time, based on knowledge from my background, lecturing in Health and Social Care. I also spent many years delivering behaviour therapy, counselling, stress management, social skills training and solution-focused programmes - in schools, colleges, and behaviour centres. I taught people how to turn off their automatic responses and how to engage healthy responses instead. I was fortunate to have these tools at my disposal, to turn off my own maladapting survival mechanisms and get healthy again, after crashing with chronic fatigue syndrome. I'm going to share everything with you now. Part one also includes a technique to access healthy states quickly, which I learnt during the relapse.

Part Two explains the missing parts to the jigsaw that are needed to stay healthy and not have relapses; the importance of living in healthy conditions and learning additional defence skills to increase our resourcefulness.

In addition to using the book, there are online videos in the *Reset to Thrive* training programme at www.resettothrive.co.uk which offer additional visual aids to complement the book. I hope this reaches people further afield who struggle with a lack of support or local government resources.

***

Now, let's take it right back to the start when I crashed for the first time. I had been living on the edge of survival for a very long time - trying to keep going, despite the onslaught my body was taking from repetitive viruses, injuries, spinning too many plates, lack of sleep and relentless disharmony. One day, I had been running around an adventure park with my daughter, followed by cleaning the house (typical full-time working mum mode). I then went out in the evening to meet friends. It started with a common cold, which is the virus that always put me in bed for days. I went to bed that night and slept for weeks. It seemed to come "out of the blue" as I had been so happy and well for weeks before, despite going through a horrible divorce. My body just completely shut down and I was bed bound and housebound for months.

As I lay in bed, unable to move, I remember thinking: "Superwoman just crashed". The smiley, "graceful swan", as colleagues called me, finally went under. I'm sure you are familiar with that scenario. Whilst it was devastating to be immobilised, drifting in and out of sleep, another part of me was unsurprised: "it has finally happened". I was diagnosed with M.E. and in those days, there was no support on the NHS, so I was extremely fortunate to have understood that the body needed to shut down, for my own protection, and knew what I needed to do to get well again. My GP was a great support, always telling me that I had "been through the mill but would recover". Looking back, I am so blessed that I had a supportive GP because I know many of my clients have not had the same support. Although I fully recovered physically the first time, I didn't change my lifestyle. I carried on as if I were invincible, took on more and more responsibilities, kept the peace and continued to be affected by people behaving badly. This led to a relapse in 2006. By now the diagnosis of M.E. had been changed to Chronic Fatigue Syndrome (CFS). Myalgic Encephalomyelitis (M.E.) means "muscle pain and inflammation of the central nervous system, the brain and spinal cord". However, there is absolutely no evidence of inflammation of either the brain or the spinal cord and so it was decided to accept the terminology used by the World Health Organisation- CFS - and standardise the diagnosis.

During the relapse, I was referred by my doctor to the newly established CFS specialist team and was devastated to be told by specialists *"you cannot recover, especially as you have had a relapse"*). Every professional insisted I had to accept the condition and learn to manage it. They told me that if I tried to fight it, I would become depressed. Yet

I became depressed *because* I was told I wouldn't recover!

Sadly, because I was referred to the specialist team, I didn't see my doctor. When I saw the GP months later about a separate issue, he was shocked when I told him what the CFS Team were telling me.

Patients referred to the team were only allowed to access group support on the NHS if we accepted "you will never recover." I had to have a number of 1:1 sessions, before I finally capitulated and said the words "I accept I will never recover" and the relief on the practitioner's face was visible, as she said, "Now we can put you onto the group support sessions." It seemed unbelievable to me, having recovered the first time; these specialists were saying to patients that you can only get support if you accept you can't recover. I really feel for all the people who were offered no hope and no method of recovery.

Everyone who was "a professional" working with CFS patients was new to the condition; they had come from other fields, ranging from Immunology to Psychiatry. However, patients referred to the CFS Team assumed they must be experts in chronic fatigue syndrome and therefore accepted what they said. CFS specialists were scrambling to work out what was going on for patients; many of whom had not recovered after many years. All NHS staff have to follow NICE guidelines so they started with the paradigm: "this is a chronic illness for which there is no known cure, therefore it has to be managed." This damaging assumption hasn't changed much since then, according to current clients. The NHS is a national treasure, and the CFS staff are invariably caring, fully committed and well meaning, but if NICE guidelines start with an inaccurate model then the outcome is bleak. It is the model that is the problem; in my experience the staff are delivering the best service they can and are often frustrated by the lack of progress. Furthermore, through no fault of its own, the NHS doesn't have the time or resources to tailor things to each individual or coach them individually through the process of recovery.

I want to share the research and solutions with people who want to recover but don't know how to or have been beaten into submission. The book offers you all the components needed to achieve recovery, and not only get your life back but learn how to stay healthy and robust. To recover from any symptoms, we need to turn on the healing system, which is currently compromised.

What is CFS?

Throughout the book I will mostly refer to Fibromyalgia (FM), post viral fatigue syndrome (PVFS) and Long Covid Fatigue as CFS, to simplify reading. CFS is the umbrella term for all related illnesses. Occasionally I will refer to PVFS and Long Covid individually when warranted.

It is likely that you, or someone you know, has been diagnosed with CFS, Fibromyalgia, Long Covid or post viral fatigue syndrome.

Symptoms include extreme malaise like having the flu, unrefreshed sleep, tinnitus, muscle pain, sleep cycle disruption and sensory overload (so that light, sound, taste, smell, or touch are often excruciating). Clearly, you will experience exhaustion; this is not tiredness, but a feeling of overwhelming heaviness, pumping heart, illness and complete immobilisation. You will have brain fog, difficulties in finding the right words, and speaking becomes exhausting. Comprehending what people are talking about feels impossible. You may be hypersensitive to food, notice your stomach can't digest certain foods and your thermostat may be all over the place, freezing or burning hot. These are all typical symptoms when the neurological system has gone out of balance and not functioning properly, and they can correct themselves when your system reverts to the healthy mode. You may also experience pain in specific joints and almost every patient will suffer from myalgia, muscle pain, all over the body.

In addition to these fatigue symptoms, people with Long Covid may have respiratory problems. There will be breathing exercises to help but do look at the online *Reset to Thrive* training programme, for specific respiratory exercises from physiotherapy and singing groups for chronic respiratory disease.

People with post viral fatigue syndrome will often experience the symptoms they had when first contracting the virus, even after it has long gone. Covid-19 and glandular fever symptoms can keep reoccurring, as does Dengue virus, for up to 6 months or longer.

Myalgic encephalomyelitis (ME) and/or chronic fatigue syndrome (CFS) is a poorly understood illness that affects approximately 250,000 people in the UK. (Nice Guidelines, 2021 p.7) It is estimated that up to 2 Million have chronic fatigue syndrome in the USA. (Sapra and Bhandari, 2021). Today, 1.5 Million have Long Covid and 45% of them report symptoms after one year according to the Office of National

Statistics (ONS 2022). According to current research, 81% of Covid 19 patients had no respiratory problems or only mild pneumonia (Zi Wu and McGoogan, 2020 p.1240). In a systematic review of 21 studies, comparing Long Covid with CFS, out of 29 listed CFS symptoms, 25 were reported by patients with Long Covid. They concluded that "Early studies into long COVID symptomatology suggest many overlaps with clinical presentation of ME/CFS." (Timothy Wong et al, 2021 p.418). Many people who contracted Covid-19 will go on to be referred to Chronic Fatigue Syndrome Clinics and suffer the symptoms of chronic fatigue syndrome. In an article to GPs in, Caroline Kamau-Mitchell, senior lecturer, writes:

> Approximately 25% of people infected with SARS-CoV-1 developed debilitating fatigue and other symptoms that met diagnostic criteria for myalgic encephalomyelitis (ME) or chronic fatigue syndrome (CFS) that continued for more than four years. So, patients with long covid who have had chronic fatigue for six months or more, together with other mandatory symptoms, are likely to be diagnosed as having ME/CFS. (12th August 2021)

> According to the World Health Organisation research (2021), key symptoms of Long Covid, include fatigue, pain, increased symptoms after physical or mental exertion, shortness of breath and cognitive dysfunction. Some patients also experience gut problems, loss of smell or taste, cardiovascular, respiratory, and nervous system problems. All the key symptoms are in accordance with those experienced in chronic fatigue syndrome, except respiratory and cardiovascular, although rapid heartbeat is also typical in CFS.

Furthermore, Nicholson (2022), identified 12 key outcomes for Long Covid: (1) Survival; (2) Fatigue; (3) Pain; (4) Post-exertion symptoms, and "functioning, symptoms and conditions"; (5) Cardiovascular; (6) Respiratory; (7) Neurological; (8) Cognitive; (9) Mental/psychiatric systems; (10) Overall physical function; (11) Work/occupational and study changes, and (12) 'Recovery'. Again, these outcomes are the same as for CFS conditions, except for respiratory and cardiovascular with some patients, where symptoms are due to tissue damage. Many people with CFS, and with Long Covid, have a racing heart and breathlessness but no physical damage.

Officially, if someone has post viral fatigue syndrome for longer than 3 to 6 months, the diagnosis changes to CFS. Women in their 40s or post-menopause seem particularly vulnerable to chronic fatigue syndrome and the same is true with Long Covid. (Costeira and Lee, 2020).

There are so many different diagnostic classifications for CFS: the Canadian classification, the London classification, the International Criteria. The London criteria includes: (1) exercise-induced fatigue precipitated by trivially small exertion; (2) impairment of short-term memory and loss of powers of concentration; (3) fluctuations of symptoms usually precipitated by physical or mental exertion; (4) symptoms present for at least 6 months, and (5) no primary depressive illness and no anxiety disorder present.

International Centre for Disease Control and Prevention (CDC) criteria for CFS includes : (1) severe chronic fatigue for at least 6 months with other known medical conditions (whose manifestation includes fatigue) excluded by clinical diagnosis; and (2) concurrently have four or more of the following symptoms: post-exertional malaise, impaired memory or concentration, unrefreshing sleep, muscle pain, multi-joint pain without redness or swelling, tender cervical or axillary lymph nodes, sore throat, headache.

CFS is a medically unexplained condition, because all the known blood and urinary tests come back negative. It is great news that tests come back negative, as it means your organs are functioning and you have no permanent damage.

The World Health Organisation classifies CFS as a neurological condition. Likewise, Long Covid is recognised as a neurological maladaptive condition; whilst a number of people do have tissue or organ damage, for the majority of sufferers the symptoms are similar to CFS and can be helped in the same way, by rebalancing the malfunctioning system. This book is to guide people how to reset the maladaptive system; it is beyond its remit to heal organ damage. With a malfunctioning neurological condition there is no evidence of damage, so neurologists are reluctant to call it a neurological illness. Muscular sclerosis (MS) is a neurological condition whereby the myelin sheath is physically damaged and there may be lesions. CFS and most Long Covid cases is a malfunction of the neurological system; there is no damage but there is a malfunction affecting our metabolism, creating sickness symptoms.

There is a reason our body was shut down; the body experienced an onslaught from a virus, operation, injury, or was pushed beyond what is reasonable and healthy. Every structure on the planet has a tolerance level, beyond which faults will start to appear, but the good news is that the body is very resilient and can bounce back. Anyone can get CFS because any body can go beyond its tolerance level. I have worked with clients from all walks of life - from surgeons, lecturers, engineers to eight-year-old children. CFS doesn't differentiate. All have the capacity to recover when they know how.

Thrive or Survive

The central premise of the book is that, for people with CFS, the body has gone into survival mode, triggering biological defence mechanisms which cause the healthy system to turn off. In this mode, your body is trying to protect you and will stay in this protective mode until it detects you are safe.

Chapter 2 will take you through current scientific research and the evidence that the body has gone out of balance, affecting automatic responses, the immune system, and the gut. In fact, evidence suggests that the body has reset itself to turn off at a low level of demand, so the smallest thing can create symptoms and exhaustion. Until you know how to change it and reset yourself back to the healthy default mode, you will stay at this low level, unable to function. Many people who had glandular fever or malaria 20 years ago still complain of functioning at only 80%, because their body reset itself when protecting them after the virus. Unfortunately, this has now become the default mode; it is the protective brain calling the shots. This will then develop patterns designed to keep you safe and avoid danger, because that is what the survival brain demands.

Knowledge is Power

Once you understand what is happening to the body, you can understand why you have symptoms. Unpredictability, lack of control and fear of the unknown, are major components of CFS and Long Covid because sufferers don't know what is happening to them; even the specialists don't know. It is very scary when you don't know if or when your body is going to pack in on you.

You would be an odd person if you didn't react like this. Even top scientists and GPs who contracted Covid were terrified of the fatigue and immobilisation. Professor Paul Garner, an epidemiologist at Liverpool School of Tropical Medicine, described Long Covid as:

> *"Like being in hell...I thought the virus had caused a biomedical change in my body and crippled my metabolism somehow. I felt insecure and fearful of the future." (Paul Garner, WebMD Health News June 30th, 2021)*

Whilst it is completely normal to feel like this, it is not useful in terms of recovery. At the moment, your protective brain, wired for danger, is staying on because it is registering that the illness is dangerous and you can't meet demands. Interestingly, Professor Garner recovered, using similar methods outlined in this book, to turn off the protective brain.

Chapters 3, 4, 5 and 6 shows you how to recover and how to manage the journey - whether you have CFS, Fibromyalgia, post viral fatigue syndrome, or Long Covid fatigue. It is a fact that a function of our higher, conscious brain is to override the involuntary, survival brain; you will therefore learn higher brain strategies to stop the malfunctioning system that is making you ill. Getting frustrated, worried, angry, or distressed, only sabotages your success and causes you to give up too soon. Everything you do from now on will be done calmly and rationally, using the higher human brain.

You know what it feels like to be lying in bed, unable to move, while fluctuating wildly between immobilisation and extreme arousal. The instinctive thing is to be terrified of what is happening but reacting to symptoms with fear will get you stuck because biofeedback from your body means the survival system will stay activated. Therefore, you need to act counter-intuitively. This is also true of respiratory symptoms.

This book is definitely *not* about making you push through; you wouldn't walk on a broken leg, so why would you do anything when your whole body feels broken, shutting down or over activated? But it is about using your body again, fearlessly and sensibly. All the resources you are going to practise are designed to activate the healthy, calm system, and to reconnect you to the world again. As you start, be mindful that any recovery or achievement is rarely a continuous upward path. I have never met anyone who has recovered without having setbacks or symptoms, even when they have evidence of recovery. Chapter 6 will explain this further and show you what to do, and what not to do, to achieve full recovery. It also refers to techniques learnt from neuro-linguistic programming (NLP) called 'Associating into Healthy States' to help you quickly reset the body, *once* you have mastered the fundamental components needed to succeed. Essentially, recovery is turning off the survival brain that is currently stuck in the ON position, meaning the healthy functioning system is compromised. It was appropriate that it took over when you needed protection, but now it is running dysfunctionally and doesn't know to turn off. To heal we have to do a manual override and get the healthy, healing system reactivated.

Part Two explains how the relapse enabled me to recognise that it is not enough to get yourself physically back to normal. To stay healthy, we have to have a healthy environment and respond to viruses, anyone and everything with healthy defence mechanisms.

Chapter 7 explains the impact of the environment on our health and how to take control of outside factors.

Chapter 8 shows you how to increase your skills set, particularly the human defence skills, in order to stay robust. You will learn how to change any habitual response that no longer serves you.

Chapter 9 shows you how to deal with viruses, symptoms, and setbacks in the future and to never get stuck again. Throughout the whole book there is research into viruses and post viral fatigue, as well as suggestions for dealing with viruses in future. This is particularly relevant and current for Long Covid sufferers, anyone with post viral fatigue syndrome and people with CFS who were affected by viruses originally.

You will know by the end of the book what is healthy and how to achieve it. You will learn to respect your body, and how to live within your healthy, normal tolerance level, as nature intended. When you are fit and healthy, the body has a fantastic capacity, so you will be able to do anything you like, as long as it is within a normal, human range. You will learn what is a healthy environment for you, and what isn't, and live accordingly.

I truly believe that too many people today have lost sight of how nature intended us to live, and this puts the body out of balance. When you get everything back in balance, when we find our niche, a healthy balance and live as nature intended, you can stay healthy.

Using This Book as a Guide and a Manual

I hope one day soon that people and professionals take it for granted that we can fully recover after chronic fatigue syndrome and Long Covid when we reset the body back to thrive mode. My greatest wish is to flag up to all professionals who work with CFS or Long Covid patients how much their beliefs, support, compassion, and reassurance impacts on our recovery. This is just as much a guide for professionals, as it is for the sufferers and their carers.

I am very aware, having had CFS and been bedridden, that reading can be strenuous and exhausting; it may be useful to start with the summaries at the end of each chapter. Read "In a Nutshell" at the end of the book, if you prefer a summary of content before digesting these topics in more detail. You may want someone to read it to you.

- If you are a Big Picture person and like to have an overview to make sense of all of the detail, then you may want to read through the book cover to cover. Then go back and slowly digest each chapter, one step at a time.
- If you prefer to start with bite-size pieces and feel overwhelmed by lots of print, then just start by reading one chapter at a time, just one section at a time.
- It would be beneficial to master one chapter before moving onto the next. It takes time and practise to become proficient at everything you need on your road to recovery. It is pointless just to read the book, as you need to be putting the recipe for success into practise.
- People who succeed the most are the ones who keep going back

to the summaries in each chapter, to refresh themselves on how to stay on track.

- Every journey begins with a single step, so just take it at your own pace and enjoy it.

Everything in this book is designed to be gentle and healthy. There is nothing that can harm you. Start by believing you *can* recover, or even being curious about what if you can.

Part One:

Recovery

Chapter 1: Beliefs

"Believe nothing, no matter where you read it, or who said it, no matter if I have said it, unless it agrees with your own reason and your own common sense. " -
Buddha

Beliefs are an incredibly important part of recovery because if you believe you can't, then you will never try to recover and if experts convince you that you can't, you will give up. But what is a belief? A belief is an opinion, but people often talk as if it is a fact. A fact is something that, by definition, we all agree on. It is a fact that there are 26 letters in the English alphabet and 12 months in our modern calendar year. They are facts because they are universally acknowledged truths. Unless there is universal agreement, everything you hear must be an opinion or a belief, just someone's take on reality. All beliefs can be backed up by evidence that supports them. Opinions and beliefs will feel very real; you may be convinced you are right; because if it feels real, it must be real. Wrong. You can have a fear of spiders and feel terrified but that doesn't mean the spider is dangerous. Likewise, when symptoms feel scary or you feel apprehensive about doing any activity, it doesn't mean activity is actually dangerous or frightening. The brain cannot differentiate between an abstract belief and concrete reality; therefore, the body responds based on what it has learnt about the situation. Danger turns on the defence systems that are already running amok for chronic fatigue syndrome (CFS) and Long Covid fatigue.

Beliefs are limiting when they negatively affect our lives, and how we want to be. Beliefs are incredibly powerful and drive our lives. People die for their beliefs or will harm others because of their beliefs. A person with a very fixed personality will stick rigidly to what they believe, even if there is evidence to the contrary, because they dismiss anything that doesn't support their beliefs. When consultants believe you can't fully recover and you have to manage CFS, they can dismiss the evidence that many people do recover completely.

I do not want to convince you that I am right and others are wrong; beliefs are either useful and serve you or they don't. We can spend a lifetime arguing about whose opinion is right or wrong but that is irrelevant. Everyone is entitled to an opinion and every belief is based on evidence, but it is better to focus on the beliefs of people who do recover than to listen to people who do not believe in recovery. When I first developed CFS, I believed I could recover because I knew the illness was a consequence of being pushed to the limit, rather than permanent damage. My GP's reassurances and belief in my recovery became my lifeline. Does your GP believe you will recover? If not, find one who does and who understands CFS. When I relapsed a few years later, for reasons that become obvious later, I was horrified that the CFS specialists were telling me I couldn't recover, and I had to learn to "manage it". They said I would become depressed if I didn't accept it. Become depressed? I was depressed at having it again and being told by "experts" there is no recovery! When I saw my own GP months later, he was shocked by the CFS Team's beliefs about recovery.

Instead of doing what I did the first time to recover, during the relapse, I started to believe what experts said; that I would never recover. They said I was lucky to have recovered the first time. Lucky? I didn't just wake up one morning and discover that a fairy had waved magic recovery dust over me in my sleep! It took faith, courage, resilience, focus, effort, mindfulness, amazing grace and belief in myself. I would tell myself: "I can, I will, and I am going to recover ". The creeping doubt, despair, and hopelessness got me stuck in the relapse. Eminent scientists and medics who contracted Covid-19 describe how frightening it is to get stuck, not knowing if they would recover. Hopefully, this will create a cultural shift in the medical world about CFS and Long Covid.

When I had the relapse, I was fortunate to find a complementary practitioner who reminded me I can recover. I did it before, so I could do it again. Everything they taught was similar to how I recovered the first time because there is a specific recipe for any success. You have to believe you can recover, do what it takes to recover, and deal with setbacks. Success is not luck; it is following in the footsteps of others who succeed and accessing information on how to recover. Healthy beliefs are an essential component of success.

The first time I crashed, I believed I could recover, and I stuck rigidly to that belief, especially on the darkest days. The second time, I started to believe that I can't recover and that got me stuck. Although I got stuck, there was always that bit of me that thought, "but I did do it before, so I must be able to do it again", and that really helped me to stay focused on recovery. I can't imagine how hard it must be for you if you didn't have a reassuring GP or evidence of previous recovery. No wonder people get stuck. Just getting the belief back makes an extraordinary difference to the body because when you replace fear with hope, you turn off the malfunctioning neurology and start to return to the healthy, healing system again.

That is the magic, not the fairy with magic recovery dust but the biology of belief. If you believe you can't recover, you will be frightened or despondent and stay in the malfunctioning protective mode. Believing you can recover activates your calm healthy physiology. If you want to look further into how belief and perception physically changes your biology, read *Biology of Belief* (2005) by Bruce Lipton PhD, a cell biologist and pioneer in this field. He explains in detail how the brain controls the body, so we need to consider the power of the brain in recovery. Also read anything by David Hamilton PhD, a pharmaceutical scientist, starting with *How Your Mind Can Heal Your Body* (2008) and *It's the Thought That Counts* (2008).

Let's start by reviewing the limiting beliefs that are commonly held, so you are better informed about the background to beliefs. Then we will look at the healthy beliefs needed for recovery. You can then make your informed choices about recovery.

Beliefs That Get You Stuck

1. The Belief that you have to Accept the Condition

Really all other limiting beliefs come from this one belief. So why do many experts and groups accept this belief?

CFS is a relatively new area of medicine, only classified a few decades ago with little previous research. Furthermore, GPs are not taught about it in training. Everyone had to start with an assumption, a paradigm. CFS is classed as a neurological condition like muscular sclerosis (MS), and so it is treated as a chronic, permanent illness. However, there is no comparable damage with CFS as there is with MS. Likewise, for the majority of people with Long Covid, there is no physical damage to organs or neurology. The CFS Service in the NHS did not exist until around 2005, so all the staff were recruited from other departments: psychiatry, immunology, and other fields. There was a lot of evidence that people didn't recover, as the first patients they saw had often had CFS for many years. No one had the answers or understood it, so people stayed stuck and this reinforced the belief that you can't recover. When specialists say "you have to accept it", what they actually mean is, "we don't have any answers and we don't know the cure". This doesn't mean there isn't a cure or a way of recovering, it just means it isn't on the NHS. The National Institute for Health and Care Excellence (NICE) Guidelines (October 2021) say there is no cure or treatment, but this needs to be understood in context. After years of pressure from M.E. groups campaigning for a medical cure, NICE will now only consider treatment that has had rigid clinical trials, including a double-blind methodology, where the administrator and the patient are unaware of what they are giving / receiving. This clearly works for the drug industry because a sugar pill placebo is made to look identical to the trial drug, but this methodology *can't* work in teaching, physiotherapy, or other therapies where the administrator *has to* know what they are delivering. As a result, NICE no longer considers them as treatments for CFS. That doesn't mean the treatments don't work, it just means they haven't met the criteria for scientific double-blind testing that is demanded by NICE for CFS, even though non-medical approaches are recommended for other conditions by the same organisation. Professionals in the NHS can only offer treatments, and get funding for treatments, accepted by NICE. They have no choice but to say there is no treatment and you have to accept your condition, because they are bound by NICE Guidelines and aren't involved in any alternative treatments outside the NHS.

At the start of a group session that I attended on the NHS when I was ill, we were asked what we wanted to achieve from the sessions. I said I wanted to recover. The practitioner was clearly shocked and annoyed, responding:

> *"I know Jan, that was an off the cuff remark. I want to make clear to everyone that this is NOT about recovery; this is about managing the condition".*

So, the experts started with the belief that you cannot recover and therefore everything they did from then on was to teach us to accept our condition. How could anyone recover in this culture? The group of fifteen people nodded in agreement with her, and I wanted to cry, not just for myself, but for all these poor souls who accepted their limitations and were grateful to hear from "experts" about "how they could manage life with CFS." Patients will naturally conform to whatever experts say, even though professionals don't understand the illness. When I did recover, nobody in the group or the group leaders wanted to know how I had done it. It is not their fault, as they are only teaching what they have been trained to teach and do not look outside the box, but progress often only occurs when we do look outside the box. Telling people they cannot recover is damaging and causes patients to give up, to conform, and to lose their resilience and confidence. This thereby contributes to chronic illness and becomes a self-fulfilling prophecy.

Our scientists and practitioners are doing their very best with what they know. They are absolutely brilliant, intelligent and knowledgeable, but they are not all-knowing in the field of CFS. At the moment, they believe you have to manage it because, at the moment, they don't have double blind tested cures. When I speak with GPs, they are fascinated to learn that CFS is a malfunction of the autonomic nervous system and all of them say that it makes sense. You do not need to get stuck anymore because there is so much research now to understand it better and resetting the autonomic system is normal practise for other conditions.

It is not just the NHS who tell us to accept it. CFS Support groups encourage us to accept the condition and help us to manage the condition. Furthermore, it is interesting that they still use the term

M.E. even though there is absolutely no evidence of inflammation on the brain and CFS has been the popular term for over 15 years. Support groups are caring and help with finances or meeting others, but they encourage you to live within the confines of the condition; their job is not to come up with treatments for recovery. Be mindful of beliefs when you speak to people about CFS and now Long Covid.

2. The Belief That Energy Is Finite, so You Have to Limit What You Do

When exertion is followed by a crash, it is reasonable to assume you should manage energy levels, as suggested in (NICE) Guidelines. Patients are told to imagine they only have so many "spoonfuls of energy a day "and therefore must conserve energy and rest after any exertion, even if they feel fine. People become terrified of using up all their imaginary spoonfuls of energy, of it running out mid-way through crossing a road, and this analogy causes them to overthink everything. This belief restricts people, keeping them stuck in the lowered threshold. The world becomes a very scary place. We become cautious about every movement, and this only serves to maintain the malfunctioning protective physiology which keeps us ill.

Patients are encouraged by Action for M.E. or the M.E. Associations to "save their spoonful of energy" for a necessary event. The reality however is that people then become anxious about doing anything, forever mindful of crashing. Life becomes a nightmare of trying to compute imaginary spoonfuls and guessing how much they have got left. It is like being on death row, waiting for the inevitable crash, and never knowing whether that last spoonful was their last one. No wonder people become over analytical, by worrying about every movement, anticipating disaster, and waiting fearfully for their finite energy to run out. Have you noticed that you have limited your activity and are more cautious about them? Do you rest before an essential appointment for fear of using up your five spoonfuls of energy and missing the appointment? Have you started measuring activity, distance, and time? If so, you are adapting to the illness. Action for M.E. believes you have to adapt, and their pacing programme teaches you to adapt.

To talk about energy as finite is an unhealthy belief. "Experts" warn us against exertion, arguing that "it is your fault you are crashing, that you are doing too much". But there is no limited battery or pool of energy to use up. The belief that we will pay for it unless we stay within very restricted limits is sabotaging success and putting fear into people, as well as making us feel it is our fault if we crash or heighten symptoms. The belief makes us live within tiny boundaries, doing very limited activity and becoming housebound, and living within the drastically lowered threshold caused by the initial crash or virus.

Action for M.E. produce guidance on Adaptive Pacing Therapy (APT) to help manage your CFS. APT is based upon the envelope theory / pacing theory and the idea that CFS is not reversible by behaviour. Patients are advised not to undertake activities demanding more than 70% of what they imagine they can do. In the APT manual, you are told to "take regular rest periods throughout the day, *even if* you feel okay." You must lie down or you will get payback." The belief is that doing almost anything will cause you to be ill because you have finite energy. The guidelines go on to say: "you will have days when you feel slightly better and at other times feel a lot worse". Note the complete dismissal that you could possibly have a good day and the emphasis on being a "lot" worse. Patients are directed to keep a diary: "the effects of overdoing it may not show up for a day or two, but your diary may help you identify what triggered your symptoms." What they mean is, you may feel great for a few days after doing an activity but our belief is you will eventually pay for it! They associate crashing on a Thursday with overdoing it on the previous Monday. This is what adaptive pacing therapy tells you to believe. Dismiss all the evidence that the body is working and only notice when it isn't, because that fits with their belief about the illness.

Energy is not finite. It is constantly created in the mitochondria, in a process called the Kreb Cycle, but production is stopped when our protective system forces a shutdown and you are trapped in the sickness loop. We need to turn off the malfunctioning system that is *stopping* production, reactivate the normal healthy system and have energy circulating again.

3. The Belief that symptoms are scary and crashes are terrifying

People who believe that symptoms and activity are scary will get stuck. They are scared when they mobilise and scared when they are immobilised. They believe, "I will be safer if I limit my life". I have met people so trapped in terror of symptoms that they literally lie in bed, petrified. They can no longer communicate, are in a darkened room, wear earmuffs and blind folds to help with the pain of light and sound and cannot be touched. These symptoms are terrifying, and I have been there. The survival system has gone on red alert, putting your senses and your whole body into heightened states of arousal. How much of the time are you scared of symptoms, worried when you are immobilised but also worried about moving?

Symptoms are terrifying, but for recovery it isn't useful to remain terrified. It is very natural to believe that life is scary, because you will have had terrible experiences and you will have had lots of evidence when you felt you were paying for having mobilised when you later crashed. I have worked with hundreds of people who were "taught to pace" and bar none, they had all become scared of doing pretty much anything.

Lyn's Story

Lyn loved dancing, and so I suggested she did a little dance, which equated to about two minutes of exercise. She was terrified and said: "I can't". I responded, "But your body feels fine just now, and your body is working, so it isn't in shut-down mode." She said that if she danced, she would pay for it tomorrow or within four days. She lived in terror, even on days when her body was working, waiting anxiously for the inevitable crash to happen. She explained that she had noticed the connection because the Adaptive Pacing Therapy told her to keep a journal to "notice these things". I suggested that this is a superstitious belief. If you believe walking under a ladder causes bad luck, you will find something eventually to prove it right. Well, what a pyrrhic victory to be proved right at the expense of staying stuck. Thankfully,

Lyn laughed when she saw another perspective, she did the little dance and lo and behold, she didn't pay for it, but she did recover.

Adaptive Pacing Therapy is encouraging the protective brain to carry on running and maintaining the "maladaptive neurological condition" identified by NICE. Sadly, it stops you using your body when it is working. Pacing is a good idea but not the Adaptive Pacing Therapy advocated by Action for M.E.. This book is about pacing yourself: doing things *when* your body feels okay; sensibly, safely, confidently, and gradually building up to increase your tolerance level. It is about adapting to healthy living, not adapting to the illness.

4. The belief that Chronic Fatigue Syndrome (CFS) can only be cured by a medical treatment because it is a real, physical illness

This is probably the most committed belief of (CFS) Associations and groups such as Action for M.E. because they are demanding a medical cure based upon the belief that CFS is not reversible by non-medical intervention. They will not support anything other than a medical cure, and in the meantime you have to just accept your condition and adapt to it. Indeed, anyone with this belief will only cite scientific research showing biochemical changes and not cite any research showing that the biochemical changes are a direct result of environmental threats causing biochemical changes in the body as it tries to adapt to conditions. Action for M.E. will only fund biomedical research and refuse to accept any other research. They have been instrumental in getting non-medical treatments removed from NICE Guidelines. It seems ironic, given that their Adaptive Pacing Therapy is *purely* based on a cognitive behavioural approach, by advising people to change their thinking about activities and recommending the need to behave in limited ways to adapt to life with the illness. At the same time, they have vehemently and successfully campaigned against any treatment that uses the *same* approach to enable recovery, such as cognitive behavioural therapy (CBT) and alternative therapies. Illogical. They are the first port of call for most people who have been diagnosed with CFS, and who are unaware of the controversy raging in this field.

The driver behind the belief that we need a medical cure is that the M.E. Association wants to prove that CFS is real and physical. This is commendable. CFS and Long Covid is real and physical, as you and everyone with CFS or Long Covid knows. With CFS, the whole body is affected; the gut, immune system, the muscles and at least twenty metabolic pathways affecting energy release, blood pressure, heart rate variability, breathing, and thermostat. People can die of this condition and 25% are bedridden, often for many years or for life. Likewise, research is showing that Long Covid is physical, affecting many of our metabolic functions.

There is no doubt it is real but having a physical condition doesn't mean that only a medical cure can treat it. This is a really important point to understand because the misguided belief about needing to find a medical cure has been getting in the way of research, effective treatments, and recovery for the patients. Hypertension, IBS, heart conditions, rashes, strokes, and pressure headaches can be relieved by non-medical intervention. Mindfulness, yoga, meditation, physiotherapy, breathing techniques and relaxation techniques have long been recognised as beneficial for health conditions. For those with respiratory problems from Long Covid, please do refer to the physiotherapy exercises, a non-medical intervention for chronic respiratory diseases online at www.resettothrive.co.uk .

There are so many illnesses that require non-medical treatments to recover. After a stroke, early intervention with physiotherapists, speech and occupational therapists is essential to make the body move again, and to recover the pathways that used to work automatically. Exercise, practise, and effort are needed for recovery. Likewise, patients, shortly after a heart procedure, are encouraged to start a minimal amount of movement to ensure the body functions properly and doesn't try to shut down. Urticaria, rashes, susceptibility to chemicals, and other conditions settle when the autonomic system returns the body to the calm, healthy position, enabling histamine levels to return to normal. CFS is the same; we need to use our body's natural healing system to recover rather than wait for a pill. Nobody disputes that muscular sclerosis (MS) is a medical illness and yet those patients are offered cognitive behaviour therapy and graded exercise therapy to improve their fatigue, which the MS Association supports.

We can influence our own bodies without medication, which is why drugs have to be tested against a placebo when the body is healing itself. Changing our lifestyle and diet has a dramatic effect on heart conditions, diabetes, strokes and other conditions. Today, the NICE guidelines are now acknowledging that painkillers are not effective for chronic pain and that the methods explored in this book are effective.

Given the widespread use of non-intervention treatments for other physical conditions, why are Action for M.E. and the M.E. Association so desperate to stick rigidly to the belief that only a medical cure or an antiviral will work? Years ago, there was a suggestion that M.E., as it was called in those days, had a psychological component, which was interpreted as "you are saying patients are imagining it or it is just a mental health issue?" It is no more a personality problem than people having irritable bowel syndrome, gut problems, tension headaches, intolerances, rashes, myocarditis, hypertension, or heart attacks and strokes, which are all influenced by overuse of the autonomic system. No wonder the CFS associations have campaigned against this and well done to them for changing professionals' perspective and understanding of the illness. Furthermore, they have funded a lot of research to prove that there are many physical dysfunctions going on with our metabolism. CFS is real and physically affects so many aspects of health. Without the campaigns from these associations, we would still be where we were 20 years ago, with no one believing we are ill. They have been instrumental in changing a medical culture and many more professionals now recognise it is a medical condition.

But in their desperation to prove it is real, they inaccurately believe, or want to believe, that only biological cures can fix it. They rigidly, vehemently, reject any evidence that treatments can come from non-medical sources and therefore sound the belief that there is no treatment or cure.

CFS associations refuse to accept that behavioural (non-medical) approaches can help recovery. This is because they believe that any non-medical treatment implies CFS isn't a physical illness. This is misleading and inaccurate. You can have a physical illness and it can then be treated with non-medical interventions. It is a physical illness that can be corrected by resetting the autonomic system, which is the neurological system that is faulty in this illness.

Sadly, patients aren't being encouraged to access treatments which can help them. People who claim to have recovered without a medical cure are dismissed by many M.E activists as frauds and are accused of never having had CFS in the first place! What a great way to win an argument and consolidate your beliefs, by dismissing and denigrating any evidence to the contrary. However, it is not useful for people wanting to recover.

CFS is definitely not imagined, and neither is it a mental health condition, but it is influenced by the brain because the brain controls the functions of the body. I don't understand why the M.E. Association and Action for M.E. are so against the concept that the brain controls the body, or that the hypothalamus in the brain has reset the threshold for people with CFS. Our recent experience with Covid-19 is showing how many very capable and competent GPs in the NHS have succumbed to chronic fatigue after contracting coronavirus. Clearly when respected medics can succumb to it, there will be a shift toward it being recognised as a physical illness, and not a personality disorder, because their word is trusted. It is wrong to believe that because the symptoms are physical, we can do nothing about it until a medical cure is found.

5. The Belief that I can't get better because I will never manage when I am better

Sadly, many people believe this belief and it means you feel doomed before you even start recovery. This is a terrible dilemma for anyone because it obviously limits chances of recovery. I would advise you to focus on getting better first, and then, only once you are fully fit and well, think about all those things. I was beside myself with anxiety about losing my job and losing our house, but I had to learn to replace fear with faith and trust we would be okay. Unless we know *for a fact* that the future is doomed, it is healthier and better to believe we will be okay; that's what faith is. Please don't let this belief prevent you from getting off the starting block. The book will guide you through how to access these health states again that were lost through this devastating illness. Part Two offers ways to manage environmental factors and how to become more resourceful after recovery.

6. The Belief that if I get back to normal life, I will crash again:

You became ill because you went over the body's threshold, what we refer to as its healthy level of tolerance. To assume it will happen again because it happened before is faulty thinking. I did have relapses again, which is why I show you in Part Two how to maintain your health forever and stop the relapses. You will be able to deal with anything and have boundaries to keep you safe and well. Life can be tough but staying ill is tougher. Better to recover and learn to stay healthy, than to stay ill.

Carol's Story

Carol had been wheelchair bound all her life because of a hip disorder from birth. She had lived a very productive life as a poet, a wife and mother. When she was in her late thirties, the medical world pioneered new surgery that would enable her to walk again. The operation was successful, but she really struggled to adapt to this new life as an able-bodied person, with all the expectations and responsibilities that brings. Suddenly, people were taking it for granted that she could do everything, and she was finding it hard to spin so many plates. Eventually, she was diagnosed with CFS, and we did some work together. After a number of sessions, she confided that she was not sure she was "ready to recover" out of concerns that all the expectations and responsibilities would overwhelm her again and she wouldn't cope. Clearly, she was running a belief that it was safer to be poorly and looked after, than to be fully fit, with all the implications she attached to this. She is not unusual in this belief; so many people with CFS have shared a similar story and sadly, many more believe it and don't seek out any remedy for recovery.

I suggested a few options to her:

- She could stay ill forever and struggle through each day but have no expectations and demands put on her.

- She could get better but then have relapses and go backwards.
- She could recover and remain fit and healthy by learning new defence skills and setting boundaries to deal with difficult situations.

Bravely, she chose to stop believing that the first two options were her only options. We did a lot of follow-up work on having a voice, setting boundaries, being assertive and improving conditions. When we spoke a few years later, she was having a wonderful life, and had a better relationship with her husband as an able-bodied person. I will always be grateful to this lady for opening up to me; had she not been honest that day, she would have just gone through the motions of the recovery training programme and would still be stuck now. Be honest with yourself and discover anything that is holding you back, and then - if you need to - speak to a counsellor or a health practitioner or go online to view my *Reset to Thrive* training programme. Eye Movement Desensitisation and Reprocessing (EMDR) therapy is also highly recommended for shifting rigid patterns, particularly as a result of trauma.

Healthy Beliefs: 10 Beliefs Needed For Recovery

1. **Believe you can recover.** As Henry Ford put it, "Whether you think you can, or you think you can't - you're right". Obviously, you can't get started unless you believe you can, or you believe it is possible. It doesn't matter how long you have had it or how different your symptoms are to others. What matters is you turn off the neurological malfunction that is creating all the symptoms downstream in your body. If others can, you can. When thousands of people have recovered, why should you be different? Be excited about the possibility of recovery.

2. **Believe it is a malfunction caused by the body getting out of balance and can get back in balance.** NICE classifies CFS and Long Covid as a neurological maladaptive condition that causes symptoms. You are going to work with the body and the body-brain to get everything back in balance, then live the rest of your life in a balanced, healthy way in future. The chapters on recovery will show you how.

3. **Believe that this is temporary and reversible.** There is no permanent damage, as there is with MS or motor neurone disease. The body needed to shut down because it was taken beyond the safe, healthy threshold and it is now appropriate for it to mobilise again. Your metabolism went into tick over mode, adapting according to unfavourable conditions, but will return to normal when you do the work to recover. Even if there are metabolic malfunctions, they will return to normal when the body's healthy system is turned on again.

4. **Believe that the world is a safe place, that I am safe.** At the moment, your protective brain is running amok, registering neutral objects as a threat. It needs the higher human brain to override it, so you are going to look for evidence that it *is* safe and appropriate to be exposed to things and to move again. This is the exact opposite of the advice given for adaptive pacing, which tells you to look for symptoms, threats and danger. Your autonomic system decides whether the world is safe or not; it automatically prepares the body for threat or nurture. Just because it feels scary doesn't mean it is scary. Stairs are just stairs, and you are going to learn to manage them successfully again. Outside is just being one step further than being safely inside, so you are going to learn that it is safe again. You will retrain the protective survival system that *you are safe* in this world, and you do not need its help.

5. **Believe it is appropriate and safe for me to mobilise.** It is appropriate to do activity gradually and safely when your body feels healthy; know you can mobilise if the body is not running in protective modes. The guide will show you how to do this. If your body feels like it is shutting down, then a sensible belief would be: it *isn't* healthy to exercise when the body is shutting down. You wouldn't walk on a broken leg, so why would you do something when it feels like the whole body is shutting down? Adopt healthy beliefs:

- Using my body is essential for recovery; when my body feels good, I will use it and be excited.
- When my body needs to rest, I will let it rest and know that it is okay and I am safe.
- I will look for evidence of times when my body is working.

Do you notice that you have been put off doing anything, after a bad experience and believe it isn't good for you? For now, believe that activity is good and know it is okay to rest afterwards, if you need to. To recover, it is important to believe that using your body is healthy. Later in the book it will become clear that your body was being shut down or activated, not by the conscious you, but by this malfunctioning, involuntary protective system. It is NOT your fault that this innate system has reset everything about the world to threat mode, but you will learn how to override this with higher functions; you have actually done this all your life, so remember that it is normal and natural to override this involuntary, biological system.

6. **Believe that nothing is scary.** Believe that everything is okay, that it will be okay to move, and to rest and to have symptoms. Later, you will learn how to stop symptoms and recover. Crashes are not scary; they are just sensations which you will then stop during this guided journey to recovery. When you notice your body is in heightened sensory arousal, stay calm and know that you are safe. These are just bizarre sensations that you are going to let pass. Whilst fear didn't cause the illness, fear will get you stuck, because it will sustain the malfunctioning adaptive system. Being fearless will turn off the survival brain. Once you understand the illness and recognise what is happening, you won't be scared, just fascinated. Likewise, it is essential with post-viral or post-infection fatigue, and Long Covid fatigue, to understand that the body is stuck in defence mode after an attack from an infection or virus; you will retrain it to get back to normal.

7. **Believe that setbacks in recovery are a normal part of the process in every recovery.** As you will discover later, setbacks are normal. They are not scary. Recovering from any illness involves setbacks and that's okay.

8. **Believe that when you recover, you will be able to manage life and deal with any situation. Because I will teach you how.**

9. **Believe it is better to be healthy, living in the big wide world, than to live a limited, safe life with CFS or Long Covid.** I believe so many people have had their spirit and confidence ripped out of them through

having this awful debilitating illness. They become disempowered and eventually conform to the new norm encouraged by "experts". When I was housebound and mostly bedridden, a colleague's wife, who had had CFS for over 15 years, came to visit me. She kindly told me, "You will get used to it and enjoy having coffee mornings with friends, rest in the afternoon, and meet others with CFS." She described how she had learnt to adjust to CFS and had a "nice little life" all the same. However, I could have wept; the prospect of spending my life like this was too much to bear. I wanted to recover, not get used to it. I was the only one in a group of 15 who did get back in the big wide world, whereas most CFS support group members I met had adjusted to a more limited life.

I wanted the choice to do whatever I liked. I wanted to live, to look after my family, to enjoy their company, and to laugh and drink with friends. I wanted to fulfil my purpose, to teach, spread the word, to fulfil my dreams, and to say no to people behaving badly or putting me down because I let them. You need to want to get back into the big, wide, wonderful world, to never lose faith and believe it is better than being safe but limited. Safe is great, but it is only the start of living. Wouldn't it be better to become confident again, empowered again and engage in life fully and believe in yourself again?

10. Believe that the illness is real, and it is physical, but that does not mean we need to wait for a pill or an antiviral cure. We know the illness is real; it is affecting up to 20 metabolic functions in the body and for many it is firing off excruciating pain in the sensory organs, in the muscles and, if you have fibromyalgia, you will experience terrible pain in the joints. Many conditions are treated with non-medical intervention. We know many illnesses require physiotherapy, occupational therapy and speech therapy to rehabilitate the patient. Stroke patients need non-medical intervention, even though it is clearly a physical condition. Likewise, we are going to work the body and use the pathways needed to get our bodies working.

A note of caution: please do not look at stories on the internet unless you know their source. There are some very unhelpful beliefs out there. There is a very small percentage of people, some of whom don't have fibromyalgia, CFS, Long Covid or post viral fatigue syndrome, who are extreme activists. The police believe there are about 50-80 of them altogether, and their names are on a list at Scotland Yard; they are a force to be reckoned with. They are on a mission to fight "the system", partly because, in America, they can only get health insurance if they are diagnosed with a medical condition. So for them, they have to prove CFS is a medical condition.

They are extremely angry towards anyone with CFS who reports that they recovered without medication. I have been the victim of this myself, as have some of my clients. The activists lambast us in the public arena if we have recovered because their belief is "if you recovered without an antivirus, you didn't have CFS and you have spoiled it for the rest of us", as I was told in numerous letters to newspaper editors. As a result, people who do recover are *very* wary of saying too much in public, in newspapers, media or online because they could be the target of vitriolic abuse from the activists. Hence, you will not see many recovery stories online. Activists crop up time and again on CFS Forums, they target any scientist who is doing research into non-medical interventions. Even the virologists who are looking at viral cures, but can't find any evidence for it being viral, are targeted because they didn't come up with the results the activists wanted! Scientists have been victims of death threats, letter bombs and abusive, threatening messages. According to Fiona Fox, Head at the Science Media Centre:

> "*Many scientists doing research on CFS were afraid to speak out in the media because of a campaign of harassment and intimidation...worst still, some had decided to leave the field completely. The terrible irony is that the very scientists who treat CFS patients, who understand how debilitating this condition can be and who are dedicated to finding effective treatments, are leaving.*" (*The Sunday Times magazine, 2013, p.19*)

It is tragic that scientists don't want to work with CFS because of potentially dangerous activists. So just be cautious of what you read, because a belief doesn't mean it is true, no matter how convincing it sounds or how vitriolic the people are. I have already had messages from clients asking not to have their stories in the book out of fear of retribution from these people. Recoverees want to stay healthy and have a peaceful life. As a courtesy, I have changed all the names in my case studies as a means to protect them.

A scanned front-page copy of The Sunday Times article:
"Scientists Under Siege" (2013)

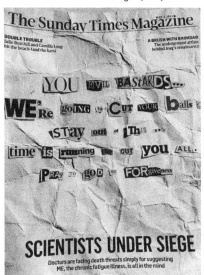

Welcome to the extraordinary world of CFS. In hindsight, I was so fortunate that, because I was so ill, I kept myself to myself and was oblivious to what was happening in the CFS world. Therefore I only focused on how to recover (the benefits of not going on Google). I suggest that you too ignore forums, negative comments and debates and focus only on your own recovery. So, the question is: do you want to believe my GP and the research that says you can recover from CFS, Long Covid and related conditions? Or do you want to believe others who say you can't recover?

If you believe you have to accept the condition, you will use adaptive pacing therapy; it won't make you better, but it will enable you to live within the confines of the illness and with acceptance you may feel more at ease, safe. In my experience the majority of people with CFS, for whatever reason, become institutionalised and accept the condition. This book is not here to convince you; it is not my job to change your mind, only to give you an alternative approach to the NHS' "no treatment, no cure" option. People who recovered listened to people who said you can get back to normal because it resonated with who they are. Believe *you* can as well.

QUIZ: See if you can tell the difference between a Healthy Belief – one that helps toward regaining your health - or an **Unhealthy Belief** that will help keep you unhealthy. These are all genuine quotes from people I encountered in the confusing world of CFS.

1. I know I will pay for it if I do too much, if not today, then next week.
2. I took five steps, so I will be able to do one more. If I can do that, I can do anything in time.
3. Symptoms are scary. I lie in bed, terrified of what is happening to me.
4. It's okay; it will pass...everything does. Stay completely calm
5. If I recover now, I should have before. I will have wasted all those years and feel dreadful that I put my family through that.
6. This is the biggest challenge of my life, but I need to do it.
7. It is better to learn how to recover, one step at a time.
8. It's okay if I rest. My body just needs to catch up with itself. Sleep is the body's natural healer.
9. Running on the spot in my kitchen means I'll pay for it.
10. It is a physical illness, so telling me to reset the protective system is rubbish.
11. If others can recover, it must be possible. I'm going to find out how to recover.
12. So you are saying it's my fault I got ill?
13. Blame doesn't help me recover; learning what it takes to recover is useful.
14. It's genetic so stop telling me I can recover.
15. What if I *can* recover?

ANSWER: HEALTHY BELIEFS: 2. 4. 6. 7. 8. 11. 13. 15.

All the others are completely understandable but are unhealthy beliefs that get you stuck; they are not part of any journey to success, so don't use them.

If you hear yourself saying anything that is not useful, stop, laugh at yourself, regroup, and remind yourself that those limiting beliefs will get you stuck. Decide to have healthy beliefs instead. For the moment, suspend any negative beliefs about recovery and be open to considering how I and many other people recovered.

EXERCISE: Copy the healthy beliefs and put them on your wall, add them to your calendar on repetition, so you see them regularly.

Summary

Beliefs are just opinions, even when they are cited by experts. The CFS world is full of conflicting opinions, distortions, and beliefs, so it is essential that you harvest healthy beliefs that enable you to recover. There is no point discussing who is right and who is wrong; what matters is whether the beliefs we have, what we think about the illness, symptoms, activity, and rest are useful and healthy. Unhealthy beliefs get us stuck.

Focus only on the beliefs and opinions of those who do recover, not on those who don't. If others can recover, so can you. Online forums are skewed toward catastrophe, because people who do recover don't want to be targeted by activists and angry people who say it is impossible to recover or that they are frauds. Keep reviewing the quiz answers and have the healthy beliefs entrenched in your mind, and be determined to recover.

Unhealthy Beliefs get us Stuck.
Healthy Beliefs enable us to be Healthy Again.

1. Believe you can recover.
2. Believe it is a malfunction caused by the body getting out of balance.
3. Believe that this is temporary and reversible.
4. Believe the world is a safe place.
5. Believe it is appropriate and safe for me to mobilise.
6. Believe that nothing is scary.
7. Believe that setbacks in recovery are a normal part of the process in every recovery.
8. Believe that when you recover, you will be able to manage life

and deal with any situation.

9. Believe it is better to be healthy, living in the big wide world than it is to live a limited, safe life with CFS.

10. Believe that the illness is real, and it is physical, but that does not mean we need to wait for a pill or an antiviral cure. You can rebalance your own body and be empowered again and recover using non-medical interventions.

Chapter 2: Thrive or Survive: The Science Behind the Illness

"If you took everything experts know about the human body, we are still only seeing the toenail of an elephant." - From a personal conversation I had with Anthony Pinching, Professor of Immunology at the Peninsula School of Medicine.

N.B. I am aware that you may not love science or have too much brain fog to take it all in, so feel free to read the bullet points below and the science summary at the end of the chapter and come back to read the rest when you feel more able.

In this chapter we will look at:

- How the body goes into survival mode if it detects threats, hardship or demands that are too difficult, like walking or stairs. Essentially, you have been hijacked by the protective system and it is malfunctioning.
- An explanation of our adaptive system and how it advances the body's survival patterns if there are threats, what are commonly referred to as our fight, flight and freeze modes.
- How over-activation of the survival systems causes illness and symptoms over a long period of resistance, as the body battles

to adapt to what it detects are harsh conditions. The ultimate phase is exhaustion and fatigue, or shutdown.

- How a lower tolerance level means you end up in a Catch 22 situation, unable to do anything without crashing again.
- How you become automatically conditioned to turn on the survival system for normal activity that you used to take for granted. This then makes us distressed, frustrated, or anxious, thus compounding the illness by keeping the protective system on alert.
- How the experience of having post viral fatigue syndrome (PVFS) or Long Covid can also make us concerned about viruses in future. This process is not conscious; it is the unconscious brain making connections about what a virus or infection now means for you.
- The need to turn off our survival mode, and instead activate the vagus nerve attached to our healthy parasympathetic system, to thrive again. This will gradually bring the lowered tolerance level back to normal and enable the body to heal.
- We need to disconnect normal, neutral activities and events from the survival system and reconnect them back to the healthy parasympathetic system and vagal nerve. By doing this, the brain relearns that everything is safe, and can mobilise again.

Chronic fatigue syndrome (CFS) is not tiredness but a complete shutting down of your body. Crashing with CFS, PVFS or Long Covid Fatigue is caused by the ultimate, ancient part of our survival brain: the reptilian brain. It is the weapon of last resort that is designed to protect you. With these illnesses, the reptilian system has taken charge, causing you to stay immobilised for long periods of time. It is not only the body that has shut down, but the brain too, so you develop brain fog and feel dissociated from life and may also experience chronic pain. The crash is the brain deciding that the body needs to shut down, for your own well-being and you are not part of that decision making.

When you have a racing heart, tense muscles, pain, nausea, or general sensory overload, it is because you have been thrown into the highly sensitive primal survival system, originally used by our primordial ancestors for looking out for threats.

It was necessary in the beginning to have the protective system look after you when you first took ill, but it is not useful when you are being stopped in your tracks for the smallest moments of exertion. You are desperate to be up and running and interacting with others, but "the issue is our nervous system- we are not making voluntary decisions" according to Stephen W. Porges, neurobiologist, and creator of Polyvagal Theory.(2015, p.12). It is registering that everything is a threat, especially when you have been reset to a very low tolerance level. Of course, the survival brain is only doing what it is meant to do when it detects you need help or need protection. But it is malfunctioning in the sense that it has become the default mode and has become over vigilant. Crucially, it is also preventing recovery.

Because of the awful experiences we encounter with this illness, the world quickly becomes a scary place. It is completely understandable to think, "If it feels scary, it must be scary". But just because our nervous system is detecting neutral events and objects as a danger, does not mean they are actual threats.

Complete shutdown or acute symptoms are a result of the body being taken beyond its natural tolerance level, either after an acute physical trauma such as a powerful infection or virus, or because of chronic, long-term physical duress and emotional / social discord. Many people with CFS will have had post-viral fatigue, but it can also be triggered by life events, conflict and demands. The illness itself, being unpredictable and scary, perpetuates the malfunctioning system which caused the illness in the first place. We now need to stop this "stuck" system and mobilise ourselves back to normality.

Researchers are trying to find the answers to what is going on for people with CFS and related illnesses. There are many scientists who focus on the individual symptoms, such as a lack of energy, and they work at a microscopic level to identify metabolic dysfunction and biological markers in cells; this is called doing research downstream. When energy production isn't working at the mitochondria level, many people then contribute this as a cause of CFS. Sarah Myhil explains this in her book "It's Mitochondria not Hypochondria" (2017). Furthermore, cell danger response (CDR) is when mitochondria stop energy production and transfer energy to defence if a threat is detected. (Naviaux 2014). This may be when there is an invading virus, infection, or gut problem. Patients with CFS showed abnormalities in 20 metabolic pathways, 80% of which were under-functioning or hypometabolic (Naviaux et al,

2016). Chronic fatigue syndrome is clearly a very real, physical illness affecting so many different functions in the body.

However, other research focuses on looking upstream to the source of the problem, causing symptoms downstream in the body. It suggests that the energy process has been ground to a halt on purpose because the body has been put into survival mode. There may be hypometabolism at a cellular level, but it starts with the brain detecting a threat and putting your body and metabolism into tick over mode. This will become clearer as we look at causes further upstream.

Research into the malfunctioning protective system shows that hypometabolism is a *result* of things going wrong further up the chain rather than the cause of CFS. I have great respect for the work of researchers in cellular biology and they have highlighted it as a biological illness, but the key for full recovery is dealing with the overriding cause. Upstream is going back to the source and getting to the root of all these problems. As Henrik Vogt and Elling Ulvestad (2016) point out in their research, metabolic dysfunction is not exclusive to CFS and to find a correlation does not imply it is the cause of an illness; they highlight evidence suggesting it is the body adapting to the environment. Indeed, Naviaux, a few years later, states that cellular changes occur *because* of environmental conditions, whereby threat can be infection or physical and psychological trauma. These changes create the sickness symptoms compatible with CFS and Long Covid. Crucially, Naviaux points out that:

> *"at a cellular level, the cell danger response cannot be turned off until the cell receives the final "all clear" signal. Until then the CDR remains stuck in a repeated loop that blocks further healing. Danger can be real or imagined...the perception of safety leads to calm. The perception of danger leads to hypersensitivity."* (2020, p.40)

This means it is the environment causing the body to adapt and change as a way to deal with threats. We will get stuck in chronic sickness and unable to heal *until* our body recognises our world is safe and returns to healthy cellular functions. We are going to make the body recognise it is safe so healing can happen and you can recover.

Nutritionists will offer a plethora of supplements and diets to try to correct the various metabolic lows in the gut and the immune system.

This is reasonable and healthy, but before investing huge sums on them, I would urge you to turn off the protective mode that inhibits digestion and get your healthy neurological system working, because it is this healthy system that enables digestion and absorption of the supplements. Otherwise they will just pass through you, and you will just have had a very expensive wee! Better to find the solution at the source than to try to resolve each individual symptom with a multitude of remedies.

Currently, scientists are undertaking the biggest research into genetics with CFS that has ever been done. (decodeme.org.uk.) and I am sure it will reveal some interesting findings. Neurophysiologist Stephen Porges, in his seminal work, Polyvagal Theory, shows how the body's defence mode makes the body go into tick over mode, immobilised but functioning at a very low level, like we see in CFS. This means that this dysfunctioning survival mechanism, by causing the body to shut down, creates the symptoms as a result. It leads to the metabolic processes underperforming, including energy production. This is what is meant by the cause being upstream: the result of biological changes being made downstream in the body.

Vegard Wyller (2009), in his development of a causal link (p.1), demonstrated how sustained arousal of the autonomic system affected metabolism and caused CFS. "Infections, which commonly trigger CFS, generally elicit a normal arousal response. Comparable arousal responses can also be elicited by critical life events and perceived chronic difficulties..long term" (p.7). Research completed by Roy Freeman and Anthony Komaroff (1997), tested people with CFS and found "patients with CFS show alterations in measures of sympathetic and parasympathetic nervous system functions". (p.357).

Furthermore, Anthony Papadopoulos and Antony Clare, endocrinology researchers, have shown that the hypothalamus, pituitary, adrenal axis (HPA) is:

> *dysfunctional in many people with CFS and associated with worse symptoms and /or disability and with poorer outcomes to standard treatments for CFS. Regarding etiology, women with CFS are more likely to have reduced cortisol levels. Cognitive behavioural therapy can increase cortisol levels and is probably the first line approach for correcting HPA axis dysfunction at present, as steroid replacement is not recommended. (Papadopoulos and Cleare, 2012 p.22)*

Here are scientists saying that a physical condition can be rectified by non-medical intervention, but CFS associations discount all evidence suggesting this. Thankfully, this malfunctioning protective system, which is something researchers know a lot about, can be corrected. We need to look at why the body is being put into survival mode.

Thrive Or Survive:
How Nature Adapts to Its Environment

Before we look at recovery, let's briefly consider how the human body functions and how it is the same as every other organism on the planet. It is humbling to remember that we are no different to other living organisms. Every living thing on earth adapts to its situation; when conditions are favourable, they thrive, grow and multiply. However, if conditions are unfavourable, they use all their resources purely for survival and then, as it struggles, it will become diseased and stop producing. Organisms don't consciously decide to adapt to their surroundings, it just happens naturally, and our bodies are the same. Adaption is an involuntary, automatic response.

This is what happens when mitochondria have a cell danger response. It thrives and produces energy in good conditions, then adapts when there is a threat, putting all its energy into fighting threats, viruses, or environmental threats such as physical or psychological trauma, and thereby leaving us exhausted and depleted.

A healthy system functions in a healthy environment, whereas the protective system goes to work when the environment isn't favourable. We all know this just by observing plants or animals around us; they are adapted to thrive in specific conditions; some plants thrive in dry, hot conditions while others thrive in cold wet conditions. A polar bear will struggle in the desert and an elephant will struggle in the Arctic. They will try to adapt but die if conditions are too harsh. It is such common sense that we take it for granted, and yet we have forgotten to apply it to ourselves.

As in nature, your healthy adaptive system functions in a healthy environment; the protective system turns on to help you cope when the environment isn't favourable. The survival system is only designed to kick in as a temporary measure until conditions improve. We need to live in a healthy environment, and if we don't, the body will automatically go into survival mode. In recent years, many people have been affected by Covid-19 and many Long Covid sufferers are experiencing terrible fatigue. Clearly any powerful virus, infection or toxin means the survival system kicks in to protect us. Post viral fatigue is when the body has been attacked by a virus, but it is still reacting as if under attack, even when the war is over. Apart from being attacked by foreign bodies, an environment can also have many other unfavourable conditions, as we will explore later.

For now, consider whether your environment is a nurturing one. Does life seem easy now or a struggle? We are incredibly resilient by nature, and are determined to carry on, even when life is hard. Chronic fatigue syndrome is such an extreme illness, and when the survival mechanism detects life is hard or frightening with the illness, our body stays in survival mode, and symptoms get worse. Sufferers unwittingly get trapped with PVFS and CFS. At the moment you are surviving, not thriving.

Hans Selye, an endocrinologist, wrote a letter to the science journal Nature, explaining how every living organism will biologically adapt to suit the environment around them. He called this the General Adaptive Syndrome (GAS) and it has had an impact in understanding factors in diseases. (1936 p.32). You will notice how much relates to CFS and Long Covid. He shows how living organisms, including human beings, go through three stages, in a bid to survive, when conditions are unfavourable:

Stage 1. ALARM: Fight and Defend. A living organism will go into red alert, pumping out all its energy and resources to deal with the hardship. For humans, this is when we are feeling highly aroused and are only able to keep going through adrenaline and other powerful chemicals that give us a temporary boost in energy. Mitochondria will divert energy to fight the infection or virus.

Stage 2. ADAPTATION: Resistance, Disease and Illness. When unfavourable conditions carry on, all living organisms go through a period of resistance. This is when the body fights to keep going, despite the unfavourable external forces, but struggles to cope. It desperately

43

tries to adapt to the tough conditions.

Whereas the body should maintain a perfect balance (called homeostasis) at this point, the body starts to oscillate wildly, tipping too far one way then trying to correct itself by going to the other extreme. In humans, blood pressure, histamines, sugar levels, and the immune system can all go out of kilter as a result.

Selye, in his 1936 paper, says that it is at this stage that humans start to become susceptible to diseases and viruses because their body is under duress. Did you notice that you became more susceptible to gut problems, sleep deprivation, and infections and viruses prior to the initial crash? If so, there is a good chance you were in the resistance stage. Humans can survive in that stage for a very long time because the body is miraculous, and life is resilient. However, you can survive but you aren't thriving.

Given that I taught the General Adaptive Syndrome, I knew, years before I crashed, that my body was paying the price for living in conditions that weren't good for me, but still I carried on, hoping that somehow the conditions in my environment would become more favourable, or I could find a way out and then my body could settle. My medical records show that in the ten years prior to the crash, I was in Selye's resistance stage, having repetitive illnesses, collapsing with low blood pressure / low blood sugars, and was susceptible to viruses and post-viral fatigue after every bout of the common cold. I had irritable bowel syndrome, a distended tummy, and skin rashes in reaction to everyday household chemicals that had previously never affected me. Unfortunately, when the medical model looks only at the symptoms, it is easy to end up with a cocktail of pills and potions to deal with each symptom, but living on antibiotics, steroids, and Imodium is not a long-term solution.

I knew it was my body struggling to adapt to unfavourable conditions and strife. It was surviving but not thriving. I believe the only reason I managed to resist for so long was because of the amazing resilience of the human body, and my children, who gave me the mental determination to battle through. It is not a coincidence that so many people with CFS have a history of susceptibility to viruses, sleep deprivation, gut problems, headaches, and skin problems. They also tend to be people who, despite what is going on, keep going without complaint. The human body is incredible, but it is also fallible if pushed too hard, for too long. Did you have any sign that the body was struggling before your body packed in?

Anyone can keep going under unfavourable conditions, but it is when the conditions are long term that problems arise. The world we live in must be sustainable.

Stage 3. EXHAUSTION. The final stage of adapting to an unsuitable environment is exhaustion. Recognise this? This is when the body has literally had enough and cannot correct itself anymore. Prolonged duress can weaken the immune system, increase risk of heart disease, and increase our blood pressure. Ultimately, the body's only defence as a result is to go into shutdown mode.

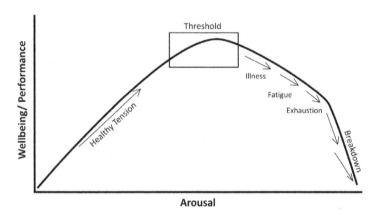

Diagram showing effects of Selye's General Adaptive Syndrome

CFS and Long Covid is the final shutdown stage, when the body has said "enough". I knew when I crashed that I had hit the final stage and whilst it was devastating for me, it was not a surprise because I taught health and care. In this sense I was extremely fortunate because I can't imagine how terrifying it was for you and others who crashed and didn't know what was happening. At least I understood what had happened to me and knew how to work with nature to correct it. You have been through the mill, your body has been shut down because it couldn't keep going under duress, so it is essential in the initial recovery to rest, rest, rest, because this is nature's natural remedy. Rest is not lying down terrified or agitated; restorative rest is when you lie peacefully and nurture yourself. Once you have rested from the initial impact, as you will learn throughout this book, you will better understand how to approach recovery and use your body to regain full health. You will live in a healthy environment and be resilient to whatever curve ball life brings. The diagram above shows what happens to the body if taken beyond its natural, healthy threshold.

What is happening within us to create symptoms?

We know that every organism on the planet has a way of detecting danger and threat, so it can adapt accordingly. In human beings detection occurs in a tiny part of the brain called the amygdala and it is like an antenna, picking up signals. Your amygdala is like a meerkat, always looking out for you.

When the amygdala detects the world is safe, it sends messages to a specific region of the brain (called the hypothalamus) that all is fine. This region of the brain manages your autonomic bodily functions, such as your sleep pattern, thyroid, thermostat, blood pressure, digestive system, and immune system. When it receives instructions that you are in a safe environment, it keeps the body running smoothly and calmly.

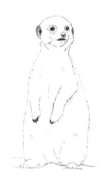

However, when the antenna detects that all is not well, it instantly sends a message to the body brain that there is a threat. It always errs on the side of caution; better to react and then realise it wasn't really a tiger than not to react, get eaten, and realise too late it was a genuine threat.

The hypothalamus controls our autonomic nervous system (ANS), allowing you to automatically adapt to your surroundings and conditions. It turns on your survival system if there is any sign of threat. This hypervigilant survival kit means you have the instinctive startle response when someone bumps into you by accident. When you assess the situation and realise it isn't a threat, you go back to normal and carry on. The diagram below may make it easier to see how what is happening upstream, in the amygdala and the body brain, affects everything in the body's metabolic functions downstream. Information streams down from your brain, telling the body to go into action.

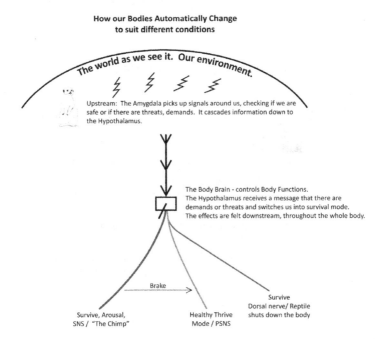

How our Bodies Automatically Change to suit different conditions

The world as we see it. Our environment.

Upstream: The Amygdala picks up signals around us, checking if we are safe or if there are threats, demands. It cascades information down to the Hypothalamus.

The Body Brain - controls Body Functions.
The Hypothalamus receives a message that there are demands or threats and switches us into survival mode.
The effects are felt downstream, throughout the whole body.

Brake

Survive, Arousal,
SNS / "The Chimp"

Healthy Thrive
Mode / PSNS

Survive
Dorsal nerve/ Reptile
shuts down the body

A healthy body is one that lives in the green track, very occasionally going into red then back again. Imbalance happens when the red track stays on too long, or when the grey track takes over to protect you. (Obviously, the tracks in your body aren't actually red, green and grey, but it's an easy way to remember them). Essentially, the hypothalamus is like the points on a train track; it flicks the switch, triggering a branch of your autonomic system (ANS), depending on signals it is receiving from your amygdala and from feedback from your body. It turns on the sympathetic system (red) if demands are too great and reverts to the healthy system (green), if demands are resolved or past. Dorsal (grey branch) is switched on if demands carry on relentlessly, or as a result of a single very powerful trauma / attack, then your energy plummets as you are shut down. Fatigue is your body shutting down. Your autonomic system is the mechanism that enables us to adapt *automatically* to situations by switching back and forth between Thrive and Survive modes. All of this is triggered involuntarily by external stimuli - you are not part of the decision making.

A Summary of Downstreaming

1. The amygdala turns on the part of the brain that controls the body.
2. This part, the hypothalamus, then turns on the adaptive system called the Autonomic Nervous System (ANS) to enable the body to automatically adapt to whatever conditions it needs to deal with. If there is a threat, it activates the red track for survival. It keeps you in thrive mode when everything is fine (green track). The grey track is activated as a last resort to shut down the whole system.
3. These processes, upstream in the brain, affect all the metabolic changes downstream in the body, which we looked at earlier with Naviaux. Today, there is a great deal of research showing how the body changes at a biochemical level.

How we get stuck in the survival states

Look back at the previous diagram and you will see that there are two defence mechanisms at play:

1. Mobilise: Fight or Flight

The sympathetic nervous system (SNS) defends by mobilising us into action and puts us into high arousal. The diagram below shows how, when demands outweigh supply, the high arousal defence mechanism turns on to pump you up and meet the demands. It is like needing to constantly jump up to touch a ceiling, but when reserves are low or we can't do it on our own, the "rocket fuel" kicks in to give us that extra surge. You will feel highly aroused and charged up. If you were a car, you would be in the high revs, the red part of the dial on your rev count. This is great for getting out of danger but very detrimental long-term.

Unfortunately, with chronic fatigue syndrome (CFS), the more exhausted you become, the less you can supply. Everyday things become more demanding. Life becomes a downward spiral, as we use the turbocharge that is already dominating us and makes us more ill.

Supply

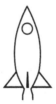

Demands

When you experience high arousal symptoms, such as feeling wired, hypersensitive to light and sound, it is the fight and flight mechanism running amok. Sensory overload is a sign that the body is on red alert, which isn't helpful when you have CFS or Long Covid. When this branch is turned on, it puts you into extreme high arousal because it wants you to mobilise. It comes on either because there is a perceived threat, such as when symptoms are overwhelming, or because your supplies physically can't meet the demands of daily activity. It will be automatically triggered if activity is a threat. Caution and anticipating disaster keep this survival system activated. As it is now malfunctioning and overreacting, it can also come on for no reason at all. The sympathetic system is a fantastic system if you must jump out of the way of a lorry but not useful if it turns on just because you have to climb stairs or walk outside. This system is often referred to as "the chimp" because it is easy to imagine the state of arousal when a chimp is in charge.

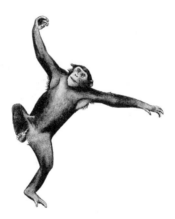

Unfortunately, it is impossible to fight or flight from symptoms, but the chimp will keep trying to mobilise you, nonetheless. Have you noticed problems with your stomach and bowel movements, sensory overload, or a susceptibility to viruses and infections? These are all associated with over-activation of the chimp mode, the sympathetic system. When you look back, you will probably recognise that you had some or many of these symptoms long before crashing with fatigue. On the previous diagram of General Adaptive Syndrome, this is "illness" before complete "exhaustion", Selye's resistance stage.

2. Immobilise: Freeze

Look at the grey track in the same diagram on how the body automatically changes to environments. When any system lives in a high state of arousal for too long, there is an emergency cut off switch designed to shut down the body and prevent it from destruction. In humans, it is the dorsal vagus nerve. It is the ultimate defence mechanism, only used as a last resort if we are about to blow the engine. To use our car analogy, in this mode, your engine has been put into "tick over "mode and you are stationary. There is nothing physically wrong with a stationary car; when you are immobilised, please be assured, there is no damage. The body will tick over, immobilised, until it is deemed safe enough for you to proceed. This is the experience of having chronic fatigue syndrome or Long Covid - it is not just tiredness or fatigue. Your body has been shut down, running at a sustainable level to conserve energy, hence the low metabolic functions we referred to earlier. The dorsal vagus nerve, attached to the calming parasympathetic branch of the autonomic nervous system, is like the fuse box in your house. When the system has been over activated, its job is to break the circuit for your safety. Your body is literally given a power cut. It is not that your "battery doesn't work "or that you can't produce energy; production was intentionally stopped because the survival brain detected that you need shutting down and it doesn't want you to be running around. The crashes you experience and the debilitating fatigue you have is because this ancient, immobilisation device has kicked in.

> "Health consequences of this state can include chronic fatigue, fibromyalgia, stomach problems, and low blood pressure." (Dana, 2018 p.17)

Immobilisation is activated when your survival system detects it is unsafe to mobilise. Interestingly, this ultimate protective system is actually part of the healthy, calm system, in green on the diagram (called the parasympathetic system). Look at the diagram on the autonomic nervous system again; the chimp (or sympathetic nervous system) pumps you up and the parasympathetic system brings you down to a normal, relaxed mode. But sometimes it brings the system down drastically, to the point of only ticking over, if that's what it detects you need. When you are being protected, it is your body doing its best for you under the circumstances. Never be annoyed with what has happened. This immobilisation system goes back to reptilian evolution, so is often referred to as the "reptile system" or "reptilian brain". You are put into freeze mode, a reptilian response to any danger.

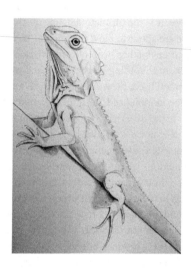

To keep it simple, it is best to think of the survival brain as being either in chimp mode or reptile mode. When you feel wired or sensitive to the environment, the chimp is in charge. The crash is the reptile kicking in.

Unfortunately, with Long Covid and CFS, it doesn't take much to give you symptoms of high arousal or complete shutdown. You are functioning at a very low tolerance level; reserves are low. This means demands outweigh supply; you struggle to meet the demands of everyday life. The tragedy of this illness is that the illness itself, exhausted of reserves, turns on the very thing that has malfunctioned: our protective defence mechanisms. Then the unpredictability, the lack of solutions from experts and concerns about what is happening to us, only feeds the survival mechanisms even more. No wonder people go on a downward spiral or restrict demands to meet their tiny amount of reserves. But there is a way out of this downward spiral, and you will retrain the body to do things healthily without turning on the survival system.

To recover, you need to get rid of all threats, so that the body knows it is safe; then it can remobilise and thrive again. You will go from hyperarousal and hypoarousal to being back in the healthy green track, your calm parasympathetic nervous system (PSNS).

At the moment, your survival brain has become hypervigilant, telling the body brain to constantly prepare the body for the slightest sign of danger. It detects you are not in a good place and struggling to thrive, so it keeps the survival system stuck ON to protect you. In effect, your body has become too hypervigilant, recording that nothing is safe. With PVFS, the virus went long ago, but the protective brain is still running, preventing the healthy, healing branch from activating anti-inflammatories. In terms of biology, you can thrive or survive, but you can't be in both modes at the same time, just as a lightbulb can't be on and off at the same time.

It is crucial to understand this on / off switch device controlled by the hypothalamus, because whilst survival systems are on, your healthy system, designed to enable digestion, healing and repair, is not functioning and therefore your recovery is impaired.

Why Can't I Do Anything Without Crashing or Getting Symptoms?

Vegard Wyller and Hege Eriksen (2009, p.2), published their research findings in the Behavioural and Brain Functions Journal and reported that there is a "change of set-point in homeostatic control circuits" in people with chronic fatigue syndrome, and so people are in sustained arousal at a low threshold of exertion. The hypothalamus has reset your threshold to a much lower level; this means you can hardly do anything before experiencing fatigue, symptoms, and illness. The tolerance level of any mechanism is the point at which it can tolerate load and stay fit for purpose. When you take any structure beyond its tolerance level, it will experience strain and breakdown. Engineers measure the tolerance level for every construct to ensure it is fit for purpose. In fact, the engineering term for overload is "fatigue" and materials become fatigued when they are taken beyond their tolerance level. Likewise, every creature is created with a tolerance level; when it goes beyond its natural tolerance level, healthy functions break down. This is consistent with what we learnt about adapting to an unhealthy environment; you become ill and then exhausted.

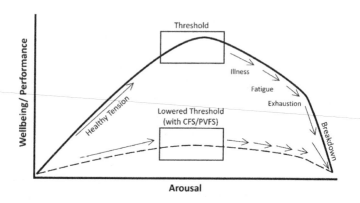

Thankfully, most people have never experienced such overload: it takes a lot for the body to shut down. Survival systems should only turn on for life-threatening events, but now, with a lower threshold, they are turning on for low level problems, such as moderate physical activity.

No sooner have you started to do something when you are shut down again. This explains why activity feels so hard. If you have been bedridden, even a tiny amount of demand reaches full capacity, so you peak and feel fatigued.

Unfortunately, so many people learn to live within the new tolerance level and become stuck. When we avoid all demands, it may be safe, but it isn't healthy to become housebound or severely restricted. I am so concerned that many people in the CFS world encourage us to live within this very limited range and make us scared of going beyond our tiny tolerance level. Indeed, the experts tell us it is "your fault if you crash because you did too much". They are working on the premise that the body cannot reset itself back to normal tolerance levels, but this is completely wrong, because many people do return to their normal tolerance levels. Even a donkey, destroyed by burden, can recover to normal thresholds if given rest and appropriate conditions.

To recover, we need to avoid pushing through when the body is in protective mode, gradually increase our tolerance levels and reset the system back to its normal healthy capacity, just as after any serious illness that has incapacitated us. Specialists and experts need to be encouraging patients to gradually reset themselves and thrive again. It is essential that you know it is appropriate to return to your natural level.

CFS, post viral fatigue syndrome (PVFS) and Long Covid are examples of some of the illnesses affected by low thresholds. No amount of wishful thinking, determination or willpower enables you to push through. I defy anyone to have these symptoms and not feel terrified, but once we understand what is going on, clarity takes the place of fear and anxiety and we can take control of the situation.

Initially, your body was taken beyond its tolerance level, whether acutely with a major infection or injury, or chronically with repetitive demands, injuries, and illnesses. Now, when reserves are low, everything is demanding: stairs, minimal walking, socialising, and then the defence system jumps in to pump you up or stop you in your tracks. When you are terrified of the fluctuations, the body will be shut down even more because the brain detects that it is not safe to raise the tolerance level. You are being controlled by the survival brain and you need to get you back into thrive mode again. Your amygdala has become over vigilant, detecting everything is a problem, and the body is being thrown into fight, flight, or freeze.

Recognise this? Do you ever notice yourself feeling cautious about going out, going for a walk, or seeing people? That's the chimp running the show. You don't want to be wrapped in cotton wool by a hypervigilant meerkat, an overactive chimp and our ancient reptile systems. You want to be thriving.

It is worth considering if our biological system may be, naturally, more easily aroused. Evidence suggests that people with CFS have a propensity to be easily aroused, and an inability to turn off the survival system quickly once it has been aroused. In the book, Why Zebras Don't get Ulcers,(2004), Robert Sapolsky, a Professor of Biological Sciences and Neuroscience, explains that a zebra will be aroused when it sees a lion, and erupt into fight and flight, but then as soon as the danger has passed, reverts instantly to a state of calm. The zebra then carries on as normal, healthily and happily. Zebras only get thrown out of the healthy, calm body for long enough to react to danger and then quickly revert to normal. They cannot anticipate danger or reminisce on past scary events that cause fear and anxiety. Sometimes, ignorance is bliss!

But humans have the capacity to think, reliving moments that have happened and anticipate danger in the future. Anything past, present, and current can then keep the body in sustained arousal. In his book, Sapolsky (2004), discusses "disorders that involve subtler undersecretion of stress hormones..these include chronic fatigue syndrome, fibromyalgia, rheumatoid arthritis"(p.15). This means the body is not going straight back into the calm, healthy state, like a zebra, but staying in the defence systems for too long. If you stop to consider for a moment, have you always been a zebra, reacting momentarily to a situation and reverting to base instantly, or have you noticed that your physiology was affected by things, and stayed affected by the lion, or other stimuli?

If our system is easily aroused and fails to turn off easily, it is little wonder that eventually the reptile brain had to kick in. To live with the chimp so regularly turned on ensures our healthy thrive system is equally turned off. It means we have a sensitive system that reacts powerfully, currently too powerfully, to our environment, like a meerkat, reacting quickly to anything that could be a threat. It could be innate, or it could have been conditioned by our upbringing and surroundings.

Also, there is a lot of evidence now that certain people are born with a less than perfect vagal brake, so it doesn't kick in early enough to prevent us from going into full-blown fight, flight or freeze mode. If the vagus brake for people with CFS is less efficient than others, it won't kick in quickly enough to turn off the aroused chimp brain and revert us to the calm parasympathetic state. You should not get thrown into the high arousal physiology for every little thing. The brake should be a highly tuned mechanism which calibrates how dangerous the situation is, recognise that "this isn't a tiger ", and put the brake on to stop your body overreacting. Like the zebra, it should let us return to a calm body once the lion has gone.

However, the brake may not be calibrating properly for people with Long Covid and CFS, so it doesn't kick in, and the system gives you full-blown responses too often. You should only feel that powerful, full-on fight and flight reaction for physical danger or complete isolation from the pack, not for walking outside, meeting people or climbing stairs. Throughout the illness, notice if your body is recalibrating things to be a big deal, when they never were before.

Thankfully, as Stephen Porges explains during an online seminar with The National Institute for the Clinical Application of Behavioural Medicine (2015), you *can* correct it because humans are evolved to consciously override the animal survival system and re-engage the healthy system. This will become obvious shortly.

How We Become Affected
by Activity during Illness

"From birth to age three, babies gain more than a million neural connections every second." (Dr Jack Schonkoff et al, 2017).

As well as having the threshold lowered and the chimp jumping in to help, there is another reason we become affected by activity. When babies make a million neural connections every second, clearly it is a completely unconscious process, and it is how we made sense of our world since we were born. You are not consciously deciding how the brain is shaped. The brain makes connections, or associations, based on the experiences we have. A child is not consciously making a million connections every second! In the same way, we are not making conscious decisions to associate one thing with another. The brain does it for us. This is important to understand for recovery. It is no one's fault that the brain made unhealthy connections when it had a bad experience; that is what it is meant to do.

The brain learns to hardwire neural pathways when things happen at the same time. It is called classical conditioned learning, or a Pavlovian response, named after the scientist who discovered that dogs started salivating to a bell after being exposed to a bell ringing, every time they saw food. Any stimulus would work: a ping, a buzzer, anything, as long as it happened at the time food appeared. The brain instinctively turned on the body's salivary glands when there was any connection to food.

This research then led to an explosion of research and how the body reacts *involuntarily* to triggers. You are (hopefully) not salivating to a bell but your body will be involuntarily reacting to triggers and experiences because this is how the brain functions. Just think how often you feel compelled to look at your phone when you hear a ping! This is a conditioned response - you didn't always react to sounds like this. You learnt that the "a ping means someone is connecting with me" and the ping makes you respond. Technology has latched onto this Pavlovian response, so you get notifications and alerts on your phone or laptop that make you respond. The trigger causes your response. You have no say in the matter; it is much quicker and more powerful than your clever rational brain. Even when you become aware that the trigger is making you respond, it is hard to resist the temptation. Resisting impulsive triggers takes conscious effort! All advertising and marketing use conditioning to make you buy their product, associating their product with feeling good, pleasure, fame, fortune, and success. To keep up with trends, their products are now associated with having a sustainable planet. You may think you are making a conscious choice, but it is your unconscious brain putting two and two together. Commerce relies on this "buy by association" strategy. Heinz did it so brilliantly with beans that they hardly need to advertise. Their slogan was "Beanz Meanz Heinz ", so every time you buy beans, you automatically associate it with Heinz and pick up their product.

It is fascinating how much our physiology is triggered by our world without us even realising. In fact, about eighty percent of how we respond is through these unconscious associations. Almost everything you understand about the world was the brain making sense of what everything means, without you even realising it was doing it. Depending on what they have been exposed to, some people learn that they can trust others, that school is exciting, that they are valued, that the world is safe and easy. People who had a different experience are therefore wired differently, based on exposure and experiences. We become programmed to respond the same way, every time, to each trigger. You have no control or choice over this, until you do something *consciously* to change the programming and make new healthy associations.

CFS and related illnesses therefore becomes a perpetuating condition, as Monique Heijmans explains below:

> "The arousal response may eventually become associated with neutral events, such as moderate activity, through the process of classical conditioning. "(Heijmans, 1998, abstract).

Neutral events, like walking and chatting, have now become conditioned to physically turn on your survival mechanism. Whilst the salivary glands are turned on for anything associated with food, the survival physiology is *automatically* triggered by bad experiences. If you were exposed to stairs or walking when you were unwell, you may have noticed the body reacting when the demand was too great.

The brain made the connection between the object (stairs) and the bad experience, so it will shut you down when you next attempt to climb stairs as a way of protecting you.

The brain has now physically hardwired stairs to your defence system through neural connections. Throughout this illness and shock, your brain learnt that you had bad experiences through these everyday demands. When you try to do anything, the defence systems are automatically triggered. Also, unpredictability and the unknown become triggers for activating the protective mode. Experts and CFS Associations see the effect on the body and encourage you to avoid the trigger, but to recover, you need to expose yourself to the trigger when the body feels okay and change the response. Thankfully, once you become conscious of triggers, you can take control, just as you can consciously decide to ignore alerts on your phone.

You are going to learn to physically disconnect everything from the chimp and reptile and reconnect everything back to your healthy parasympathetic system. The process for change is:

1. Expose yourself to movement and activity *only* when you are in a good state, and firing off healthy responses, so that you have good experiences and success with this activity.
2. These good experiences and successes mean the unconscious brain makes the connection that everything is safe and manageable.
3. When everything is safe and manageable, they will be hardwired again to the healthy branches. Triggers will then activate the healthy green branch. Use the healthy pathways and lose the protective ones.

When you activate the healthy parasympathetic branch, you can thrive again.

How the Autonomic System Affects the Immune System and Viruses

"Ongoing stress...has a tendency to suppress the immune system, thus setting the stage for infection. Fibromyalgia and chronic fatigue syndrome, a condition believed to be closely related, are examples of the inflammatory response gone awry. A sluggish HPA axis has been implicated not only in asthma but also in arthritis, fibromyalgia, chronic fatigue syndrome." (*Bruce McEwan and Elizabeth Lasley, 2002 p.100*).

The body should function in perfect balance, networking amongst all the vital systems. When the autonomic nervous system goes out of balance, and is skewed toward defence and survival, it causes imbalance in the rest of the body. In unfavourable conditions, the autonomic defence systems are aroused and then illnesses occur in the resistance stage, as highlighted by Selye (1936). The gut and immune system will be compromised when the body goes into survival mode for too long, as McEwan and Lasley explain above.

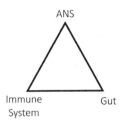
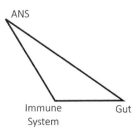

Your illness may have started with a virus or infection, or at least it was "the straw that broke the camel's back", causing the immune system, autonomic system and the gut to go out of balance. Once out of balance, the protective system goes on overdrive and the healthy system doesn't function properly, thereby creating a vicious cycle as all the organs and metabolisms are affected, making recovery from viruses, gut problems and other conditions harder. It would be useful here to consider if you were already hitting the healthy threshold before you were so badly hit with the virus? We will consider the physical, intellectual, emotional, and social overload in later chapters, but for now, were you functioning at full capacity, with few reserves in the tank to cope with a virus?

It is more than likely that before post viral fatigue syndrome (PVFS) or Long Covid, you had been pushing yourself too close to the tolerance level, with little reserves to fight the powerful virus. This is characteristic of Selye's resistance stage, where you were functioning well on the outside, but the body was compromised. People from all walks of life are becoming more susceptible to viruses when reserves are low: Long Covid, PVFS and CFS do not differentiate between socio-economic groups.

Immunologists who research CFS / ME have shown that people with CFS re-activate the immune system, increasing inflammation and cell danger response. As Philip Schreiner and his colleagues note:

> "In conclusion, HHV-6 reactivation in ME/CFS patients activates a multisystem, proinflammatory, cell danger response that protects against certain RNA and DNA virus infections but comes at the cost of the mitochondrial fragmentation and severely compromised energy metabolism." (Schreiner et al, 2020 p.201)

As mentioned previously, Papadopoulos and Cleare (2012) have shown that the Hypothalamus-Pituitary-Adrenal (HPA) axis in CFS is "out of balance, functioning inappropriately, affecting the gut, the immune system and our metabolism"(p.22). This means when the autonomic system is out of balance, our immune system will not be working efficiently either. This supports Cleare (2004) who also stated that "HPA axis changes can be reversed by modifying behavioural features of the illness, such as inactivity, deconditioning and sleep disturbance" (abstract). This is reassuring.

Sapolsky's previously referenced text, *Why Zebras Don't Get Ulcers*, offers a plethora of findings from researchers, showing that stressful conditions make us susceptible to viruses. He writes that scientists have discovered that the "autonomic nervous system sends nerves into the tissues that form or store the cells of the immune system" (Sapolsky,

2004 p.144) and the immune system has receptors which are particularly sensitive to hormones released from the brain. This means that the brain and autonomic nervous system affect the immune system. Selye showed that the thymus gland of mammals atrophied when subjected to unpleasant conditions. Modern research indicates that long term stress affects our immune system in so many ways, including inhibiting antibodies, inhibiting the anti-inflammatory function and affecting the ability of the T cells to fight foreign bodies. Any chronic unfavourable condition, whether physical, social, emotional, or mental overload, will produce the same results. Some of the stress chemicals released will stop the immune system suppressing inappropriate cell division, thereby leading to tumours and cancer. (McEwan, 2002).

The sympathetic nervous system also suppresses immunity during stress. McEwan refers to research showing "stressful periods have been shown to precede the onset of immune- related disorders, such as MS and juvenile diabetes. People who are more psychologically stressed are less resistant to respiratory infections that cause the common cold". (2002). When the red or grey track is on, inflammation increases. You cannot be in the healthy track and in survival modes at the same time; the deactivated green track cannot produce anti-inflammatories, which are needed to heal the body after infection.

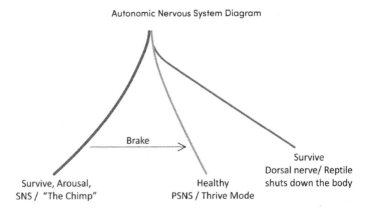

Autonomic Nervous System Diagram

Brake

Survive, Arousal,
SNS / "The Chimp"

Healthy
PSNS / Thrive Mode

Survive
Dorsal nerve/ Reptile
shuts down the body

During the first stage of being infected by the virus or foreign body, the immune system goes into action and inflammation increases as cells rush to the site. However, as Sapolsky explains, acute stressors boost the immune system and put it into action, but if the stressor carries on for more than an hour, sympathetic activity and stress hormones, particularly glucocorticoid, have the opposite effect and suppress the immune system.

Suppression is fine if the problem is resolved, as the immune system just goes back down to its normal baseline point.

> "It is only with major stressors of longer duration, or with really major exposure to glucocorticoids, that the immune system does not just return to baseline, but plummets into a range that really does qualify as immune-suppressing. For most things that you can measure in the immune system, sustained major stresses drive the numbers down to 40 to 70 percent below baseline." (Sapolsky, 2004 p.155).

Consider whether you were already hitting the threshold before succumbing to viruses, and whether you are still hitting the threshold now.

In a controlled study, Sheldon Cohen, a neuroendocrinologist, exposed volunteers to the common cold, rhinovirus, after housing them in various conditions at the Common Cold Unit of Medical Research in Salisbury, UK. In their research, they found that "that stress is associated with the suppression of a general resistance process in the host, leaving persons susceptible to multiple infectious agents". (Cohen, 1991 p.612). Infact susceptibility was nearly three times greater under stress, irrespective of age, gender, personality or if living with other people.

"Prolonged stressors more than a month-long, that were social in nature, provided the greatest risk", according to research by Janice Kiecolt- Glaser and Ronald Glaser (1991), who were pioneers in demonstrating how marital strife and bereavement can undermine the immune system more than physical burden. We are social creatures, and our health is clearly influenced by people around us. Social discord affects emotional and mental overload as well. Although there is now substantial evidence showing that long term stress or overload can impair the immune system and increase the risk of illness, the immune system is so complex, and scientists still don't know exactly how it works. However, as you recover, it is important for you to access healthy support and avoid hostility as much as possible.

To reiterate, when the chimp or the reptile survival mechanisms are on, the healing parasympathetic nervous system is deactivated and therefore cannot produce anti-inflammatories. The survival system has taken over control of your body and is in default mode. Inflammation causes multiple symptoms, including pain, heart rate increase, breathing problems, tightness of chest muscles, rashes, and fatigue. Long Covid is being categorised as an autonomic dysfunction just as CFS is an autonomic malfunction (NICE Guidelines). This means that instead of being in the parasympathetic system that enables anti-inflammatory function to restore the body, the adaptive system is stuck in survival mode. Reflect whether your autonomic system was running in the healthy "green track" or the "red track" prior to infection? (See the previous diagram.) In hindsight, was your lifestyle reasonable, sustainable and healthy? Now, with this illness, are you feeling like life is tough and see symptoms as a problem, or are you relaxed about recovery? It is normal to be devastated but it isn't useful for resetting to thrive mode.

Often a powerful virus causes the body to go into shock and get stuck. Epstein Barr, herpes and varicella- zoster (which causes chicken pox and shingles) are latent viruses and they flare up when the immune system is suppressed, often due to stress. Have you ever noticed any markers from glandular fever, such as swollen glands or swollen eyes, which flare up years after having contracted it? It is not a coincidence that they flared up at times when you were stretched to your max. How do these clever latent viruses know to come out of hibernation? According to the work highlighted by Sapolsky (2004), the virus DNA "is sensitive to elevated glucocorticoid signals, and when the levels are up, that DNA sensor activates the genes involved in coming out of latency"(p.170). This means when stress levels are high, the virus is activated. Once you have a latent virus, it is important to live a sustainable lifestyle, with reasonable demands and keep your supplies high.

THRIVE: Achieving Our Goal to Thrive Again

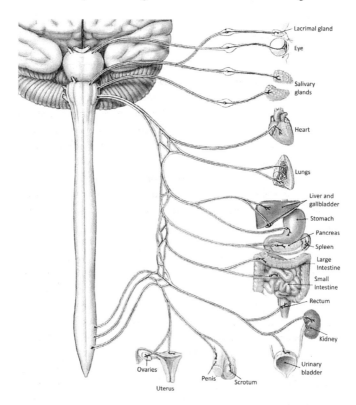

Diagram of the Vagus Nerve

We should be living in the parasympathetic system because it enables all our organs and metabolisms to function normally and keeps us healthy and thriving. It is the system needed to heal the body, repair, and recover.

Attached to the parasympathetic system is the ventral vagus nerve. Vagus means wandering, because this nerve weaves its way from the brain through the rest of the body, connecting all our organs. It is a two-way system going to and from the brain: into our ear to detect auditory tone, into our facial muscles to detect tension, into our vocal cord to detect the tone and pitch of our voice, into our chest cavity to connect with our lungs, chest muscles and heart, and finally into our abdomen to connect with our digestive system and organs. It detects if you are functioning normally by picking up your tone of voice, gestures, and other feedback from inside the body.

The vagus nerve physically connects your facial expression and tone of voice to your lungs and heart. If you have become vigilant, and are looking for any threats during illness, the vagus nerve automatically changes your breathing and heart rate accordingly. It is therefore *crucial* to check that your facial expression and tone of voice are appropriate for recovery. A frightened tone will set your heart racing and affect your breathing- not good for embarking on an activity. You can now see why it is so important to activate this nerve, as it affects every organ in the body.

When survival systems are stuck on, the healthy system is deactivated, turning off functions in the body; no wonder you aren't thriving. In his seminar for the National Institute for clinical Application of Behavioural Medicine (NICABM), Porges, the creator of Polyvagal Theory, argued that "the issue is [when it comes to] our nervous system - we're not making voluntary decisions" (Porges, 2015 p.12). This means that it is essentially your nervous system that is reacting to stairs, activity, and events, not the conscious, rational you. Our feelings about the world around us is based on which physiology was triggered initially. Do you notice that your body reacts powerfully to symptoms and crashes? This is not your fault. You have no control over your initial autonomic responses, but I will teach you how to override the primal response using our facial expressions, tone of voice and posture to reactivate the soothing parasympathetic system. The animal defence brain relies on non-verbal signals to communicate meaning, so you will become a master of non-verbal signals. You will also engage higher brain activities and higher social defence systems to inhibit the lower mammal and reptilian systems, which is causing malfunctioning neurological illnesses such as CFS and Long Covid. It is completely normal to override lower systems. During a discussion with Ruth Buczynski at the National Institute for the Clinical Application of Behavioral Medicine, Porges says the human "autonomic nervous system has a whole component of voluntary input. We can...change our breathing, change the motor tone to our face...with chanting, with mother's lullabies, with motherese speaking – [our tone of] voice is important" (2015 p.5).

So based on the science, the way to recover is to sensibly build up to normal thresholds, make healthy connections with neutral events, engage the human brain to recalibrate events and reactivate the healthy vagus nerve that enables healing and recovery. This can be achieved using vagal activation exercises and using healthy resources, which you will learn throughout the guide. You will focus on how to thrive, rather than focus on protecting yourself from anything that has become hard.

Reflecting this fundamental need, my online training programme is called *Reset to Thrive*, and you will find online training videos to complement this book at http://www.resettothrive.co.uk

Summary

Humans adapt to circumstances just like any other living organism; if the circumstances are favourable, then we thrive, but if life is hard, then the body will go into survival mode. In CFS and Long Covid, the protective, survival brain is dominant. It was appropriate in the beginning for your body to shut down, but it should now turn off. The body can only be in survival mode or thrive mode - it cannot be in both at the same time. What is happening in the amygdala affects everything in the body. When the amygdala has learnt that everything is hard or too demanding, it instructs the hypothalamus, the part of the brain controlling the body, to turn on survival defence systems. All living organisms go through three stages of trying to adapt to unfavourable conditions. In humans:

1. **Mobilisation**. The body goes into red alert, firing off the mammalian defences to put us into fight and flight.
2. **Resistance**: This is the stage when the body desperately tries to adapt to challenging circumstances. All the systems go into overdrive, but it is unsustainable. Eventually, the body will start to suffer, and become more susceptible to illnesses, diseases, gut problems and viruses.
3. **Exhaustion**. The final stage of survival is exhaustion, when the body is so fatigued that it has no more reserves to call on. You hit the threshold and crash. At this point the body shuts down. Chronic fatigue syndrome and fatigue symptoms with Long Covid is the final stage of exhaustion.

Survival is controlled by two different branches:

1. The Sympathetic Nervous System (SNS) is for mobilisation, represented in red on the autonomic nervous system (ANS) diagram. Also called the mammalian or chimp system, it puts you into arousal for fight or flight and shuts down any normal functions that are not needed, such as digestion, reproduction, restorative healing and repair.

2. The dorsal vagus nerve, represented by the grey line on the ANS diagram, immobilises the body, and puts it into freeze mode for its own protection. You are safe, but just ticking over. This is the reptilian mode.

Neither the highly aroused chimp or the immobilised reptile defence systems are meant to be used long term - it is unsustainable, and they malfunction, causing imbalance and illnesses.

Thrive mode is shown in green on the diagram and it is the system you are meant to live in all your life, unless you are about to fall off a cliff.

Your chimp and reptilian systems are controlling your body. Evidence suggests that people with CFS and Long Covid have been hijacked by the survival system, after acute or chronic overload to the body, causing all the symptoms of high arousal or shut down that you experience. Metabolic functions are compromised as a result of having the protective system running inappropriately, which means your healthy system is turned off.

This is why the illness is called a malfunctioning neurological condition, or maladaptive; it is *adapting* the body to prepare for threats, even when there are none, and it has taken charge. Thankfully, you can override this base system.

Throughout the illness you had bad experiences when your threshold had been lowered, so the brain learnt that activity is dangerous and so kept the protective system on. Most of how we function is through this involuntary, conditioned learning; the brain makes new associations about neutral events/triggers and how the body needs to respond. Furthermore, when demands outweigh supply, the body naturally fires off the chimp, to pump you up to try to meet demands.

Based on the science, the way to recover is:

- To eat healthily and sensibly, reduce your fat and refined carbohydrate intake, as they overload the body and activate the protective system.
- Build up to normal thresholds without help from the chimp.
- Re-establish healthy associations with neutral events by using healthy resources, such as focus, confidence, resilience and serenity.
- Engage the human brain to recalibrate events and practice healthy resources to reactivate the healthy vagus nerve.
- Do gentle physical exercises to kick start the vagal system again and enable all the organs and metabolisms, including energy production, to function properly again.
- You will override the malfunctioning adaptive system that is stuck in survival mode, and you will make the vagal system work again.
- Everything you do from now on as you work through the chapters is based on what it takes to reset back to thrive.

Chapter 3: Recovery. Reset From Survive To Thrive

"A journey of a thousand miles begins with a single step." - Lao Tzu

You have already started your first steps to recovery by understanding what is happening to your body and therefore how to correct it. Take your time to go over the previous information before moving on to the rest of our toolbox for recovery. We are going to:

- Increase our energy threshold back to the normal range by doing reasonable, achievable activity and exercises. Defence systems only kick in if demands are perceived to be too much.
- Make the world safe and manageable so the body naturally switches back to the thrive branch of the adaptive system.
- Disconnect activities from the protective system by eliminating threat, fear and anxiety. Reconnect neutral events back to the healthy parasympathetic mode, which heals the body and lets it thrive.
- Engage the higher brain to override the lower survival instincts.
- Notice when you are functioning normally, in the healthy green track, the parasympathetic nervous system.
- Stop perpetuating the condition during chronic fatigue Syndrome (CFS), post viral fatigue syndrome and Long Covid.

Let's just quickly review how you may be stuck in a loop during recovery from a virus, like Covid-19 or from overload, before learning the tools to break free.

Right now, does it feel as if life is hard? Does it feel as if you are surviving, not thriving? Your body will respond accordingly, and if you feel like life is hard, then you will be stuck in a never-ending loop, as shown in the diagram below. Remember, Naviaux explained that at a cellular level, the body gets stuck in a sickness loop until the environment is safe and free from threat.

At the moment your survival brain isn't getting the signals that you are safe and confident. Do you ruminate on the symptoms, on crashing and get anxious about symptoms happening again? This is hardly surprising given that adaptive pacing therapy, recommended by CFS associations and professionals, tell you to limit activity so "you don't pay for it." They mean well, but what you get when you receive a message that activity is dangerous is a patient who naturally becomes fearful, cautious, and protective. The amygdala keeps a record of all threats, and the body stays in defence mode, affecting metabolic functions.

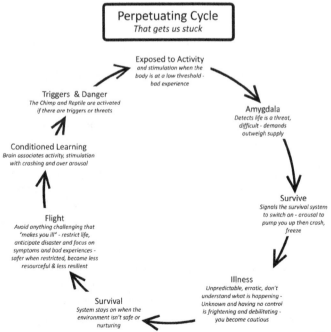

Perpetuating Cycle
That gets us stuck

Exposed to Activity
and stimulation when the body is at a low threshold - bad experience

Triggers & Danger
The Chimp and Reptile are activated if there are triggers or threats

Amygdala
Detects life is a threat, difficult - demands outweigh supply

Conditioned Learning
Brain associates activity, stimulation with crashing and over arousal

Survive
Signals the survival system to switch on - arousal to pump you up then crash, freeze

Flight
Avoid anything challenging that "makes you ill" - restrict life, anticipate disaster and focus on symptoms and bad experiences - safer when restricted, become less resourceful & less resilient

Illness
Unpredictable, erratic, don't understand what is happening - Unknown and having no control is frightening and debilitating - you become cautious

Survival
System stays on when the environment isn't safe or nurturing

Here is a case study of Sarah, one of my clients. She initially developed
PVFS, but this developed into CFS:

> *Sarah was a super fit horse rider when she developed
> post-viral fatigue syndrome after getting glandular fever.*
>
> *She had been getting up at 5am to care for the horses
> and look after her children, then riding after work. She had
> volunteered to start work an hour earlier because of staff
> shortages, so was getting up even earlier and becoming
> exhausted. She increased her workload because she felt she
> couldn't let people down and yet, in focusing on others'
> needs and not her own, she became susceptible to viruses.
> She was highly conscientious and so good at caring for
> others, but not herself. After getting Glandular Fever, she
> was desperate to get back to normal, so as soon as her body
> was able to walk about, she went back to doing normal
> activities, as a full-time physiotherapist and busy mum to
> three children. She struggled off and on for months and
> was then diagnosed with PVFS, which led to CFS.*

Whether it started with a virus or another reason, really challenge your
values, your beliefs and assumptions about your use of terms such
as "having to", "got to", or "should", and how they determine your
workload. Listen out for those words in your head. What patterns do
you run? Resilience and keeping going are excellent traits, but not good
when your body is struggling and you ignore it. Sarah was the enthusiast
who spun lots of mental, social, and physical plates in her life, but was
often unaware of her limitations. Enthusiasts don't appreciate that
every organism has a threshold; rushing around, they don't know how
to be truly relaxed. If this was you, there is a very good chance that
to meet demands, you were running on empty, and didn't have the
reserves you needed to fight off a powerful infection or excess load. I
have worked with many sports people, enthusiasts and teenagers who
were floored by a powerful virus because, at that time in their lives, they
were already living to their max, which is unsustainable. Teenagers,
young people, and menopausal women are particularly at risk because
the body is using a huge amount of energy in transition, and hormones

influence the immune system. When enthusiasts are hit hard with a virus, they tend to be impatient about getting better, run before they can walk, then crash, become devastated, and consequently sabotage their recovery.

You are not going to push yourself from now on. Let's look at some saboteurs and learn the art of being patient.

Saboteurs

1. Vicious Cycle after Viruses or Initial Illness

If, like Sarah, you are driven by the notion that you had to get back to work or responsibilities, you will keep crashing. Furthermore, you may have gone from being the invincible busy person before the virus to becoming fearful about not getting better. These responses prevent natural recovery.

All your life, you had viruses and got over them but this time you don't. You took it easy for a while, then tried to get on with life, but this time it doesn't work, and everything becomes a struggle. You have no idea what has happened to you; the unpredictability, shock and powerlessness fires off the survival system. Having no solutions is terrifying for patients, as patients with CFS can vouch for. You become concerned about what will happen if you do things and devastated when the body packs in again. Whether the protective autonomic system was running prior to contracting the virus or not, evidence shows that when they are activated by the illness, recovery is prolonged.

It is easy for a vicious cycle to emerge when your threshold has been significantly reduced by the virus (diagram below). You try to get back to normal when your supplies are depleted and the threshold is lowered; no sooner do you do something and the protective system kicks in, causing more symptoms and fatigue/ shutdown. When the sympathetic nervous system (SNS) is on, the vagal system that produces anti-inflammatories is compromised. Activating the protective system increases inflammation and all the symptoms associated with that: pain, fatigue, virus or flu symptoms. This scenario sets up a cycle of continually going beyond your threshold, having to rest, perceiving rest as a problem, and then not knowing what is okay or not okay to do the next time.

Concern at not recovering or getting back to normal then creates threats and anxiety concerning your job, finances and responsibilities, thus compounding the activation of the survival systems. People start to be concerned about what will make them crash again. Uncertainty also means people use various strategies at this point; having never experienced anything like this before, everything is trial and error. Hence, people try and err often.

One strategy is to increase protection by reducing activity and become more limited or housebound. They try and finally give up trying to recover. The other strategy is to courageously keep trying but get frustrated, anxious, or devastated when the body won't recover.

Neither of these strategies are useful and get you stuck. Why? Because both strategies focus on threat and create anxiety or fear, turning on the very system that prevents anti-inflammatories from kicking in and additionally suppressing the immune system. When supplies are low and demands are high, the body bridges the gap with the chimp and our rocket fuels. We keep the system running in a perpetual cycle. This is nobody's fault; anyone who is desperate to get on with their lives will naturally be frustrated, anxious or depressed when they aren't recovering, and they don't know what is wrong with them. Defence systems were necessary initially to protect your body, but now they are perpetually running inappropriately and causing symptoms because they detect a threat.

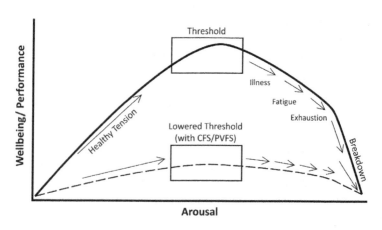

The upper threshold shows what happens when we go beyond the healthy threshold. The lower curve shows how the hypothalamus has reset the threshold to a lower level for CFS and post viral fatigue syndrome (PVFS). You now hit the lowered threshold just by doing very little exertion.

2. Conditioned Responses

> *"I believe that we can unwittingly reinforce, as Pavlov has shown, the dysfunctional autonomic tracks in the brain set up by a virus long gone." - Prof Paul Garner, Web MD(2021) Epidemiologist, who suffered from Long Covid and is now recovered.*

Through no fault of your own, the amygdala learnt that normal activity is scary; basic activities like stairs, walking, and socialising all become intimidating because you had a bad experience when you were exposed to these things at the start of your illness. Remember, the brain automatically makes associations and neural connections, just as when you automatically respond to the ping on your phone. Neuroscientists use the phrase "What fires together wires together" to explain the Pavlovian response. Healthy neural connections and associations would be:

Trigger or activity = can do = confident = competent = healthy calm physiology.

When you got ill, you had symptoms and had a bad experience at the same time as doing stairs, moving, or walking. The brain then connected all neurons for activity to your sympathetic system and dorsal nerve- the chimp and the reptile. From then on, they automatically fired off when exposed to activity or any other trigger (stimuli). Unhealthy new neural connections and associations would be:

Trigger or activity = can't do = distress = survival systems turn on. Symptoms continue.

Professionals, CFS Associations and patients notice this connection, and patients are then told to avoid the activity and be cautious of them. This is wrong. You have to reconnect normal function to the healthy system by recording positive experiences in your everyday activities, and not avoid life.

Through negative conditioning, you become trapped in a downward spiral, a negative loop, with the body constantly having to adapt to threat, and becoming more ill, immobilised, and exhausted in the process. The malfunctioning defence system is staying on because it detects you are not safe.

Conversely, the people who push through and boom and bust become devastated by crashes and setbacks because they fear they aren't recovering and that they will stay sick. Setbacks activate the protective system, affecting cellular response, heart rate, breathing, inflammation, symptoms and physical shutdown.

It happens completely unwittingly because it is an unconscious process. Your brilliant brain is making sense of the world and making connections for you. Most of the time, your brain is running programmes in autopilot and controlling the body automatically, without you having any say in the matter.

Once you become aware of what is happening, you can override automatic responses. In the book, *Psychoneuroimmunology* (1991), Robert Ader describes how your brain, hormones and immune system are forever in communication with one another and influencing one another. Nicholas Hall and Maureen O'Grady (1991), psychoimmuniologists, likewise went on to prove that behavioural intervention, "such as relaxation and guided imagery, self-hypnosis, biofeedback training and autogenic training...increase the stickiness of white blood cells, as measured by saliva and blood tests".. This means the immune system can improve when we consciously use exercises to fire off healthy hormones and activate our healthy vagus nerve. We have much more control over our bodies than people used to think, and therefore we can influence recovery and not accept the outdated, unhealthy beliefs that we have to manage CFS or post viral fatigue syndrome. The same is true for symptoms of Long Covid, where there isn't evidence of physical damage to organs.

3. Emotions get you Stuck

Whether it started with a virus or not, having fear and frustration will turn on the survival system, thereby turning off the healing system. Furthermore, while your body needs to build its tolerance, any demands can tip you over the threshold. In her published research, Dr Candice

Pert (1997), a neuroscientist and author of *Molecules of Emotion* explains that the molecules of emotion, or neuropeptides, are in constant communication with the immune system. Her research suggests that people under stress are more susceptible to viruses, whilst people in love fill the receptors with oxytocin, and block viruses from entering. We know from research, cited in the science section, that immune cells have receptors for stress hormones and other emotion peptides. Likewise, receptors for molecules of emotion affect healthy functioning.

That's the power of emotions on recovery. I can't stress enough that emotional stress and distress has a powerful impact on the body when it is already calibrated to shut down for anything that is too much for us. It is natural to have an emotional response when alerted to a problem; to combat this, we should solve the problem, or accept it with serenity. If we do not do this, the brain gets into a loop, noticing problems and having emotional responses. To investigate this further, read *The Brain That Changes Itself* (2007) by Norman Doidge. This unhealthy looping leaves you trapped in a never-ending cycle of sickness.

Furthermore, depression changes chemicals in the brain, making solution-focused much more difficult, so a large part of recovery is learning how to deal with emotions. Distressing emotions are natural and essential, but they are not useful for making rational decisions during recovery and for activating the healing vagus nerve. The body has enough to deal with and your reserves are low, so it doesn't need the added pressure. Your facial expression, your tone of voice and your breathing are all being fed back, via the vagus nerve, to register your emotional state. If you shallow breathe from the chest and tighten your chest muscles, it will send out stress chemicals to get you out of what it detects must be a dangerous situation. You can't run from a virus, so turning on ancient survival systems is pointless and counterproductive. Here is an example of how quickly emotions and negative associations get you stuck. A young man I have been in contact with called Ben wrote the following on a Long Covid Forum: "I went out for the day on Wednesday but had crushing fatigue for two days after; I obviously did too much and paid for it."

Within three weeks of contracting coronavirus, Ben, normally a fit and active 30-year-old, became frightened of crashing and was almost totally housebound. That is how easily the protective system does its job; it made the connection, "indoors is safe and outdoors is dangerous".

Notice also how our focus is crucial; Ben was dismissing the fact that he felt well for a whole day, and only focused on the crushing fatigue, meaning he only saw threats, got emotional, and therefore received further protection from the survival system.

Becoming Better

Reflect whether you are in thrive or survive. When a malfunctioning survival neurology has become attached to everything you try to do, it will sabotage success. When we are ill and reserves are low, the world is full of difficulties, so survival stays on to help you meet demands and protect you from doing anything threatening. I have met hundreds of clients who were stuck for years because they thought they were doing the right thing, by being cautious and avoiding situations that affected them. Recovery happens when you start to make your world safe by doing things that are safe, and exposing yourself to triggers when you are feeling able, capable and competent. It happens when you start associating confidence with activity. Remember, the body can only heal and thrive when conditions are favourable and safe. We need to break the circuit, STOP the survival brain running amok, and retrain the brain to make healthy connections with everything in our world. You are going to reconnect activity to the healthy system again. Like an electrician, you are simply going to move the wiring from one circuit to another, from the survival circuit back onto the healthy vagal system. You will re-cover your steps to recover.

You are going to gradually increase your threshold back to normal range. There is no magic tool to measure tolerance levels and energy, so start by taking baby steps and expect to get it wrong sometimes and that's okay. Everything from now on is OKAY because you are going to make the brain register that your world is nurturing, even though you still have symptoms. Stroke patients and people in rehabilitation units still have symptoms but gradually return to health and activity.

Do ensure your world is appropriate for recovery; if you are living in an abusive or unpleasant situation, you need to seek help urgently and read the chapter about unhealthy environments.

This is a story about how quickly we become programmed for survival.

John was 25 years-old when he developed chronic fatigue syndrome:

> *"I became anxious about doing anything and it was recommended that I do adaptive pacing, to conserve energy and avoid the crashes. Seeing people was exhausting, so I restricted seeing people to five-minute slots and could only see three people a week. Within weeks, I became housebound, and all of this happened within a few months of being diagnosed. I realised one day that my world had become so safe and so small that it felt I was living in a tiny bubble, away from the real world. Safe is such a powerful, instinctive feeling but I didn't just want to be safe, I wanted to live. Once I spoke with Jan, gradually I learnt to make a bigger world to be safe in. At first, I conquered just two steps outside the door and rejoiced! My world was getting two steps bigger! Over time, I increased the size of my physical world, one step at a time. Then, when I felt okay, I saw a friend and didn't set my timer but said I would stop when I had had enough. I had such a lovely time with my mate, and he left after 20 minutes. Even though I had to lie down when he left, I was ecstatic; my world was getting bigger and more fun, more normal. Over time, I practised expanding my world by turning recovery into a game. Of course, I had setbacks, but I focused on all my successes and accepted it would be trial and error. I know if I hadn't chosen fearlessness over needing to be safe, I would still be housebound today."*

Choosing to be fearless and to recover into an uncertain world may seem hard at first, but it is much less hard than staying stuck with sickness, and being safe in a cocoon that becomes infinitely smaller.

The Battle of the Brains

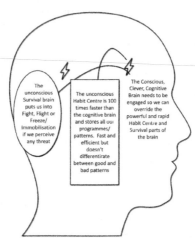

On the diagram, notice that a main function of the higher, human brain is to turn off and inhibit the survival brain and the habit centre. When we activate the clever brain, we deactivate the malfunctioning protective brain. Furthermore, when we engage higher brain activities, we activate the healthy vagus nerve and return to the normal, healthy state.

The survival brain and habit centre run automatically and unconsciously; you do not consciously choose to turn them on. They are triggered by things in our environment. Only the higher brain is conscious and can actively choose how you want to respond. You are going to learn how to turn off the survival brain and get yourself back into the healthy body again by turning on your higher brain.

Habits happen a hundred times faster than your conscious brain, so you will also learn to override unhealthy habits with the conscious brain. The thinking brain may not get off the blocks first but when it does, it is brilliant and powerful. To recover, you will turn off the malfunctioning systems using your higher brain. It is a completely normal process that you have done thousands of times. We teach children to stop being overly impulsive by training them to develop their conscious, cognitive brain and self-regulate. In the same way, we need to push the pause button when we notice instinctive responses from the lower brain, and allow the slow, brilliant brain time to engage and take control.

Traffic Light System:
Always stop and think before proceeding

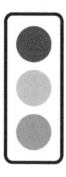

Stop. Pause to give the Higher Brain time to kick in.

Think. Engage Rational Brain. Decide consciously how you want to be instead.

Proceed In a Healthy State

By following this procedure, you will automatically return to your healthy parasympathetic mode as the conscious brain recognises that, even though you may still have symptoms, you are safe.

You are going to consciously turn off danger, turn off the chimp and the reptile, and revert to normal. You have switched from one mode to another hundreds of times in your life and you will do it again for recovery. Using the following diagram, consider the processes you go through when you notice traffic coming as you prepare to cross a road:

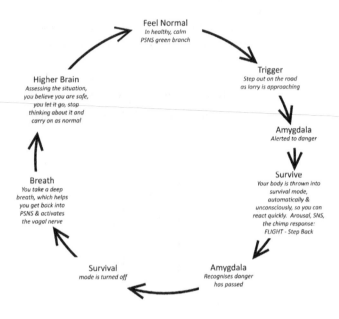

In this scenario you stopped the protective circuit. You consciously turned off the defence system by engaging the higher brain to assess you are safe, thereby returning to a normal, calm mode, and carried on.

It is completely normal to break the survival system loop and carry on. You have done it thousands of times in your life when someone bumped into you, or you spilled red wine on the carpet. You actively stopped the startle response and took control by engaging your conscious brain, assessing the situation, and letting go of the incident.

From now on, you need to know you are safe, thus enabling the body to revert back to normal again. You will use all the resources in this chapter to get back to normal. As Scott Peck said in his classic book, *The Road Less Travelled*, (1978), "whatever you truly value, you have to give it your time". So often we just don't dedicate our time and attention to the things that really matter. For now, commit time to recovery and focus on your own well-being. You will help others when you are back to being strong and healthy. Take time to master the tools for recovery. Most of the tools you will have used many times in your life, so we are just going to apply them for recovery.

Commit to doing the exercises to learn the right way to travel forward and practise being healthy again, then gradually increase your threshold back to normal.

If You Don't Use It, You Lose It

The more you use neural pathways in the brain, the faster they fire off and become the dominant, first response. When we don't use the pathways, they slow down and stop firing off because the brain and the body have to be worked. We need to make sure we are using the healthy pathways and stop using unhealthy channels. Throughout the illness, you will have been running unhealthy neural connections, but the healthy pathways are always there; they are just not being used and therefore aren't firing up. Today scientists equate the brain to being like a muscle. When you use them, muscles become stronger and if you don't use them, they deteriorate and become weak. The same happens to neural pathways.

Imagine a mountain path that is so well-trodden and overused, we can see it from miles away. Then one day, someone puts a barrier across it to stop it being used. Consequently, we use a better pathway that we had forgotten about. Gradually, as it is no longer used, the old path grasses over and disappears. The newly used track now becomes clearer and quicker to run because it is used more and more. The well-used track becomes the dominant track.

Like the mountain path, it will have been a long time since the healthy pathways were travelled along. The protective pathways have been overused, ingrained, and are always firing off first. You are going to stop using these unhealthy pathways that are physically hardwired to your survival systems because they are not useful. Let them disappear. When you notice the body reacting, just as it does in our example of seeing a threat from a lorry coming, you are going to stop it, recognise you are safe, revert to the calm state, take a breath, and stop anticipating disaster.

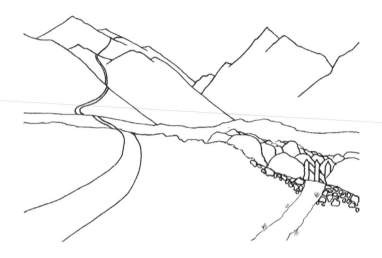

You will then proceed safely, fearlessly and use the healthy pathways. The brain loves repetition because that makes the pathways stronger and faster, automatic, and habitual. You will retrain the body to be healthy when doing activities and be at ease when you anticipate doing something. Remember red, amber, and green = stop, think, and proceed.

EXERCISE: Draw the mountain track, closing off the old paths that the chimp and reptile ran amok on. Re-open the healthy path and commit to using it, practising healthy resources. Pin it up on your wall or fridge to remind yourself to work your brain and use your body.

Summary

- If you expose yourself to neutral events in a poor state of health and therefore have a bad experience, the brain learns that this activity is dangerous and too demanding. It hardwires that event to your survival system. You do nothing to make this happen; conditioning is a normal process, just as salivary glands turn on when you are exposed to food. This means, through no fault of your own, the unconscious brain makes your body react negatively to normal activity. Your survival system becomes triggered by everything.

- You can then, unwittingly, get stuck in a vicious cycle of increasing immobilisation.
- Emotions get you stuck and affect all the parts of the body because receptors for emotional chemicals are spread throughout the body. Distressing emotions mean the environment isn't nurturing and the protective system stays on, preventing recovery. Furthermore, if you don't control emotions, they will prevent the conscious brain from engaging. We need the conscious brain to override the lower, instinctive, and automatic brain.
- The body will naturally readapt when it recognises you are safe whilst completing everyday activities and tasks.
- The brain is like a muscle, so you need to use healthy pathways and stop using unhealthy connections. If you don't use it, you lose it.
- It is normal to inhibit the survival instinct and you have done it all your life, so do it now for recovery. Do your traffic lights if you have been startled or shocked by any situation.

Chapter 4: Fearless Resources for Recovery

"Neurons that fire together, wire together." - Donald Hebb, Neuroscientist

We know that viruses such as glandular fever, Swine Flu, Influenza and now Covid-19 can have a powerful impact on the body. It can take 3-6 months to feel completely normal after glandular fever, and they are saying the same, if not longer, with Long Covid, so patience is key. You will need to learn to become as serene as a Buddhist monk and have the patience of a saint. In the beginning, rest and sleep are essential; whether you were hit by one of these viruses or crashed through the tolerance threshold another way, initially you need to rest. Sleep as much as you can in the beginning because sleep is your body's natural healer. You will do it with serenity and acceptance. The FEARLESS approach in this chapter will show you how to do it the right way. Get rid of all expectations of when you "should" recover; just know you will and follow the process for healing. Imagine your only job is to get yourself better.

During initial recovery, as you lie in bed, close your eyes, and notice how you are giving all the energy to your immune system, giving it a chance to deal with the virus or onslaught you have been through. Notice how lovely it feels to be looking after yourself and giving yourself time to heal. Surround yourself in a warm cosy bubble. You are safe, and you are getting over an illness; be grateful you are not living in a war zone. Give up all thoughts and concerns.

Feel proud of yourself for putting yourself first and saying no to everything else, knowing you will heal quicker. If you notice you worry about letting people down, be assured that most people are compassionate and reasonable. You are ill, and it can't be helped, any more than if you cancelled because you had broken your leg or had cancer. If people aren't reasonable, you probably don't need them in your life and will learn how to approach them better, later in the book. Life can go on without us - everything and everyone can wait.

Let go of all pressures and expectation from others; you will get back to work and back to the family or business quicker when you stop putting demands on your already depleted body. We are not indispensable, and if you died tomorrow, work would find a solution, so it is not true that you "have to" get up quickly. Other people can rally around and plug the gaps while you recover and stay recovered. Better that you get back to 100% now, rather than return on 80% and then need to take time off again.

When you feel able to mobilise, even a little, you are going to use the acronym FEARLESS to remember what we need to be doing. All the FEARLESS resources are the strategies used by your higher brain to turn off basal survival instincts and are connected to the healthy thrive system. You cannot be stoking the chimp and the reptile modes when you approach recovery like this. Once in the healthy state, you will then use the body appropriately. Become familiar with one resource before moving onto the next.

During my relapse, I was terrified of ending up bedridden and immobilised for life; I can promise you that fear gets you stuck. This is why you are going to replace fear with all these healthy resources that demonstrate you are safe and nurtured and don't need protecting.

FEARLESS

Focus.

Excited, enthusiastic, healthy emotions. Encouraging yourself to succeed.

Adapt. Your body will naturally adapt to a healthy environment, where nothing is a threat.

Resilient and Rational. Get back up again and keep trying.

Love and Kindness. Caring for yourself.

Emotionally detached. Be mindful of anything that feels threatening or upsetting.

Serenity, amazing grace, and gratitude.

Seeing Things differently. Perceive everything is safe, so the body naturally settles, and you can disconnect your survival mode to triggers.

Use Nonverbal Signals
to Get the Message Across

Nonverbal signals are critical for resetting the body. As Porges (2015) says during the NICABM seminar, "our social engagement system - face, voice and prosodic features - enables us to change our physiological response". How wonderful that we can change our malfunctioning physiology by engaging muscles in the face, ear, and body!

The brain is more animal than human and still relies more on nonverbal signals (NVS) than on words to understand what is going on. Your non-verbal signals account for 93% of the feedback communicating to others and back to your own brain, so really focus on your NVS as you follow the strategies for recovery. They are crucial for recovery because facial expression and tone of voice feedback to the animal, protective system whether you are safe or under threat. As Porges explains, "The cues that we are giving with our face are really manifestations of our physiology" (2014, p10). Turn off survival mode by always checking that your facial expression and tone of voice are appropriate, including when you practise FEARLESS skills.

Every part of you needs to be authentic and committed. When you want to stop the body reacting or stop running bad habits, you will say, "STOP, that's enough" in a firm way, so your auditory system can process the instruction. This is the red on the Traffic Lights system. Your voice will sound like you are giving a firm, calm instruction to the chimp or reptile, expecting it to stop. You will never shout or be frustrated because that arouses the chimp even more and makes you feel worse. Everything is about control, compassion, and conviction. Practise how you would say "stop", or "that's enough", as if you are telling a child or a friend who is in a bad state. Would you shout at them? Of course not. You would say "come on, that's enough" with conviction and warmth. Practise that same tone, expression and posture that you would use in those kinds of scenarios.

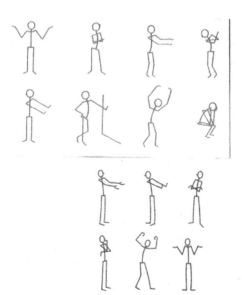

Figure 2.4 Some postures with clear meanings (from Sarbin and Hardyk, 1953).

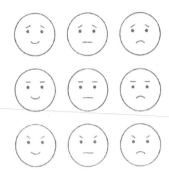

Which gestures and expressions show calm control in the diagrams above? Ensure your tone of voice, facial expressions and gestures and posture reflect the healthy states you are going to practise.

This is not a race. Be mindful that it is the tortoise who won in the end. I have seen so many people go on courses for recovery because they want a quick fix, or some kind of magic wand to make them well, then get frustrated if they aren't instantly better. Within three weeks of doing any training course, most of the information is forgotten, unless you keep revising what you learnt. Your healthy parasympathetic system is connected to FEARLESS resources, so use them to fire off the healthy mode, even though you still have symptoms and feel ill. You are going to practise being healthy again.

People who recover quicker have the FEARLESS acronym recited in their heads or pinned up, so whatever they are doing, they remind themselves to be consistently FEARLESS. Read and practise, one section at a time.

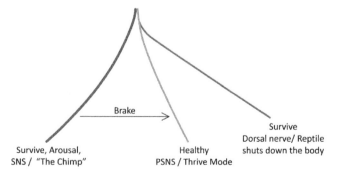

The F in FEARLESS is for Focus

Focus on what you want, not on what you don't want. As with any major illness that left you bedridden or debilitated, your protective brain is checking if you are safe enough to take initial steps and mobilise again. It is focused on threats and using this information to put you into the red or grey track on the autonomic nervous system (ANS). To get to reset to thrive mode, you are going to consciously focus on when your body is doing okay, getting better, or starting to thrive.

Neuroscientists have long recognised the power of attention processing and use refocusing as the primary tool for change, because the body adapts according to what environment it detects it is in. If you look at the world and only focus on disasters, your body will feel low or threatened. However, if you focus on how magical nature is, your body feels uplifted. This isn't imagined; your body physically changes when you perceive the world in a certain way. The world hasn't changed but your focus has, and that affects your body. Selye recognised how organisms adapt to surroundings and called it the General Adaptive Syndrome (GAS), which we looked at before. Scientists are now able to show how the body adapts, at a cellular, mitochondrial level, to the environment.

We achieve when we focus on what we want, not on what we don't want. A sports person will fail if they only focus on their failures, and you will get stuck if you only focus on failures and anticipate disasters. It may seem obvious to say that we need to focus on recovery to recover, and yet, it is very likely if you have CFS or Long Covid, that you are focused on symptoms, on analysing risk, and the disastrous consequences of completing everyday tasks. You are actually focusing on the very thing that you don't want, and the protective system is getting stuck, maintaining symptoms.

Do you notice when you feel better, or do you mostly notice when you don't feel good and can't do things? Become aware of your language. Do you say you have symptoms "all the time"? Really? All the time? Do you focus on evidence that you can do things?

Here are quotes from people with Long Covid on social media forums:

- "My body is constantly vibrating inside; there are so many symptoms, and I feel so alone in this whole scary process."

- "I am so scared of what is happening to me. My heart is pumping; I feel buzzing all over and get rashes. I feel so fatigued and am now housebound because I crashed for five days when I tried to go out. Is anyone else getting these symptoms?"

When you look at forums, the majority of the comments are focused on the symptoms. Being focused on symptoms is entirely normal, especially when no one can explain them, but it is not useful for recovery. Contrast those quotes with these ones from other Long Covid patients I found online:

- "I have completed my first two weeks back at work. I am not quite over it, still get a burning chest, on and off and slept solidly for 11 hours, two nights in a row! Hang on in there, it slowly gets better. "
- "Many more mountains to climb but overcome one. Chest X-ray is clear - Hurrah! Just wanted to share the hope."

Clearly, these people are focused on recovery, even though they still have symptoms.

EXERCISE: Using a notebook over the next few days, jot down all the things you think about. Do you think about the symptoms? Or do you notice symptoms? Or do you look for any signs of symptoms if you do any activity? Why are you cautious? Just become aware how much you focus on the illness, past, present, future and how it impacts on you.

When you do this exercise, you will be amazed by how much the protective brain is focused on problems. It is not your fault, you have been taken hostage by the chimp and reptile who, after a bad experience, become fixated on any sign of danger. This is what happens after any trauma; we are programmed for survival, and it will always dominate.

However, it is not useful for the protective brain to take over your focus. It has literally shifted your focus from noticing you are safe to looking out for danger, because that is what it is meant to do. Once it takes control, it switches your focus and looks for all the signs that you are not okay. It is trying to protect you by making you notice all the dangers and avoid another bad experience.

CFS Associations and Action for M.E. encourage you to focus on danger by advising you to be cautious. They ask you to keep a diary to notice when you crash, or when you don't feel well, and to look out for an activity you did four days ago that "caused" the setback now. They ask you to focus on problems. The amygdala registers those symptoms and activities are a problem and prepares you for fight or flight. You can't run away from or fight symptoms, so the problem increases. Your body may feel churned up, wired, hypersensitive, or in pain. When fight and flight doesn't sort the problem, the reptile brain kicks in to shut down the body as a last resort, causing immobilisation and sickness symptoms.

Furthermore, when we focus on problems, the emotions automatically turn on. This is entirely normal and it is meant to happen, but not useful if we get stuck in a loop. Do read the brilliant book, *Molecules of Emotion* (1997) by Dr. Candice Pert, to understand how emotions are chemical reactions in the body and can cause harm if triggered too often.

So you need to focus on the right stuff, noticing when you are safe and functioning. You are *not* going to pretend that you don't have symptoms, but you are going to search for normality and have a healthy focus. Remember, what you focus on is what you get, so you want to notice when your body feels better, feeling okay. There will be exercises later in the book for dealing with symptoms. In the beginning, look for any sign - no matter how small - of healing or energy, then you will start to find green shoots of recovery everywhere.

When I was completely bedridden, I had to look for the tiniest signs of progress; I noticed one day that I awoke early from a period of continual, regular sleep. Then I noticed that I was more alert when I had been drifting in and out of deep sleep. I couldn't lift my head and then one day I could! That became my focus, looking for anything that suggested that my body was healing. Of course, the progress wasn't sustained, and I would fall back into a deep sleep, but the focus was on noticing when I was better than at my worst. This gave me evidence that my body could recover. In the beginning, all recovery is intermittent, but it builds when we notice the right stuff, minimal gains, and stop obsessing on the illness. You only need one piece of evidence to notice change, to notice progress, so hang on to every tiny sign of improvement. How exciting that just making a shift in one area can have such a profound effect on your body. We are all agents of change; we can train ourselves to focus on what we want, and in this case, on recovery. Let's role model people who focus on the right stuff; if they can, so can you.

Elite sports people and people who achieve in their field have trained their minds to be utterly focused on their goal. They are not distracted or pay attention to things that are not useful for achieving their goal. Additionally, sports commentators use slogans such as "the player is utterly focused", "in the zone", "on track", '"oblivious of anything else", or "has his eye only on the ball". Focus, to succeed. In the book, *Will it Make the Boat Go Faster?* (2011) by GB Olympic medallist Ben Hunt-Davis, he talks about staying focused. He explains that no matter how many times the practice doesn't go right, you have to stay focused on the fact you can. Even on days when it doesn't feel like you can, you focus on the fact that it is possible and on what you did achieve.

Your goal is recovery, so focus on recovery and health. Pay attention to when you are okay, not on signs of illness and disaster. All success follows the same pattern, no matter what the goal. Don't focus on the end result because it will feel daunting. To achieve your goal, focus on your successes one step at a time, and accept setbacks, but do not let them be your focus. You know you are ill; you know you have symptoms, but focusing on them won't make you better, only worse. Here are some examples of how my previous clients utilised this strategy:

Sandra's Story

One of my clients, Sandra, had been completely bedridden for many years since contracting glandular fever as a teenager and was in a very poor state when I first met her. She insisted she didn't want to start her journey of recovery in bed, so was lifted onto a chair. A determined lady! On the first day, she managed to get out of the chair unassisted and we walked into her garden. When we returned, she was quite emotional, explaining it was the first time in 15 years she had been in her garden. After the training programme, she said she didn't want any follow-up appointments for a few weeks. She was utterly determined and focused, and had numerous setbacks, but clung onto the moments when her body did work. She constantly reminded herself that she could stand up from a chair because she had proof that she did it, that she can walk in the garden, because she had evidence that she did it before.

Her mantra was, "If I did it before, even once, I can do it again". Within four months she was fully fit, won Student of the Year doing an online course, and then went to college the following year. She now runs her own business, is married and very healthy. If she can, YOU CAN!

Bob's Story

One of my most humbling moments in my career was working with a 34-year-old client who had sustained a brain injury after a kite surfing accident and had been paralysed for two years. He was in a rehabilitation centre, being told by the experts that he would never walk again. He was released from rehabilitation and transferred to a care home the day I met him. Bob was a very rational man, a lecturer in engineering, and he rationalised that, as his spine wasn't damaged, he just needed to get the brain working again, to make it send messages to the limbs. He was determined to walk again, despite the odds. One day, he moved a finger on his right hand for the first time. He said, "If I can move my finger, I can move the rest of my body". He was utterly focused on the fact that he could move. This one piece of evidence became his focus, and his mantra was, "I can, I will, I'm going to".

With the help of the work we did together, and working with a brilliant physiotherapist, Bob took his first step. He then took a step, unaided, and gradually learnt to get his body working again. Last time I saw him, he was running up the road and was entering a charity race. Despite setbacks, he never lost his focus. I remember later asking him if he ever felt like giving up because he had so much evidence that, apart from his finger, his body was paralysed. He looked at me as if I were mad and said, "What would be the point in that? I just need to focus on what I can do".

Humbling and brilliant. To this day, he is an inspiration to me, and he can be your inspiration too. What is your mantra going to be?

What We Need to Focus on for Recovery

1. One Step at a Time. Let's start by taking it as a given that you want to recover, and that is your goal. Now put that goal somewhere off into the future, just as any Olympian does with the gold medal. You will get there when you do the work today. Focus on the small steps you can do today, not on the big goal. Take it one step at a time.

EXERCISE: Whenever you notice that you feel well enough, notice how you can move and focus on putting one foot in front of the other; the endpoint is out of sight, out of mind. You are just taking one step at a time. Focus on how amazing it is to be able to walk. Your body never forgets healthy, patterns, so write down the evidence that your body isn't completely immobilised or forever struggling with pain. Focus on how far you have come, and not on how far you need to go. If you are bedridden, notice when you can move in bed, lift your head or arm, or can get to a toilet.

If you think of how far you still have to go, it will feel overwhelming, and you may give up. People who achieve say. "Just put your head down and get on with what you need to be doing right now; don't focus on the next thing on the list". Only focus on how well you achieved that step, and then achieve the next one. Simon Reeve, the TV adventurer and presenter, had his life changed by being given one simple piece of advice: "If it's difficult for you, just take it slowly. Take things step by step". In fact, he called his autobiography *Step by Step* (2019). Recently, he said he still lives by that advice, taking life step by step.

Life has been difficult for you, so break things down into tiny achievements, and focus on recovery, one step at a time, even if there are setbacks.

2. Focus on Yourself. Put your health first and give yourself time to heal. You need to value your recovery and commit time and focus on it. You may notice that you spend a lot of energy thinking about other people's stuff, so refocus on recovery and trust they will be okay. If you had sepsis or were in Intensive Care, someone would have to take over looking after things, so it is possible. You are ill and need to focus on getting better. Ask for help from wherever and massively lower your standards. I can't imagine my house was cleaned properly for a very long time, but we survived! Prioritise.

Additionally, if you notice a limiting belief creeping in here, such as "I can't ask anybody to help", then really challenge that belief. What would happen if you weren't there? What would happen if you asked? So many people who get CFS are people who didn't tell others they were struggling, they didn't put their hands up and ask for help or demand help, so do it now, because changing this pattern is part of well-being. Part Two and the online training will show you how to express needs. Focus on finding solutions. If recovery is your number one priority, you will do whatever it takes to recover. Show people the evidence that this is a very serious illness, and that it is not simple tiredness. Show them the book or the online *Reset to Thrive* programme to help them realise your body is physically shutting down and you need time to recover.

3. **Focus on anything other than your illness.** When you pay attention to the chimp or reptile, you give them power. Stop. If you notice you are brilliant at looking for symptoms, you are focusing on the wrong thing. What you focus on is what you get. Focus on what you want, not on what you don't want. You know you have symptoms, so you don't need to keep checking.

Practise getting outside of yourself and focus on what is around you. Mindfulness is becoming aware of your surroundings and becoming an objective observer. Look up at the sky and notice everything. If it's raining, look for the rainbow. Be childlike again. If indoors, focus on something that takes your mind off yourself, whether it is music, cleaning, reading, writing, or watching a programme. Nurture your creativity and get absorbed in art, drawing or writing. Anything to take your mind off the saboteurs, symptoms, body checking and looping on thoughts inside your head. You will know what works for you and it is fascinating to notice how the body adapts its physiology according to whether the activity is joyful or a chore. Research into chronic pain recognises the power of distraction; the body doesn't register pain nearly as much when it is absorbed in other things. You naturally engage the healthy branch of your autonomic nervous system when you do things that are nurturing but feel worse when you force yourself to do a chore that isn't nurturing for you. (Moseley, 2018).

EXERCISE: A great technique is to take photographs, either with your phone or camera. A camera with an eyepiece viewfinder is best as it makes you focus only on what you are seeing. It is the essence of focus, a tunnel vision of what you want to capture. Notice how you feel when you are absorbed. Your body settles when it is focused on healthy things and not looking for threats. Also, watch nature through binoculars to become fixated on surroundings.

Jane's Story

> Jane was so good at body checking that even when her body felt fantastic, she said, "Oh, but I still notice a bit of pain in my toe". I laughed and asked, "How is it possible to dismiss the fact that your whole body is feeling great now, when it had been in so much pain before, and you only focus on the ache in your little toe?" But of course, that's what the brain had got into a habit of doing - looking out for any sign of illness. Once Jane laughed at the chimp and switched focus, she went on to make an incredible recovery. If you notice you are one of these people, then be amazed how your survival brain has become so fixated and dominant. Then be determined to look for any sign of well-being.

4. Focus on being normal. This is the essence of what we want. You want to be back to normal; so notice when you do things normally. Normal is living in the calm, relaxed parasympathetic mode, so notice whenever your body feels relaxed. You don't need to be doing anything; you may be sitting in a chair or lying in bed and your body feels relaxed. Hurrah! That means your body is working in the healthy mode, and not using the chimp or reptile modes. When you move around, are you taking it for granted you can, doing it without thinking? Normal is when you do things in autopilot when it is effortless, unconscious. If you are doing anything with fear, trepidation, or anticipation of disaster because you are focused on danger, you are not behaving normally. Notice when your body is working and, in that moment, you are healthy and back to normal. It may not last, but you are focusing on when you have evidence. It is not about what you do, it's how you feel when you do it.

Only ever do anything when your body feels it can and never push through. You want to hardwire activity and movement to being safe and successful so the autonomic, adaptive system switches to thrive mode, not survival mode. So many people walk, but spend the time measuring their paces, scared that they are doing too much and will suffer for it. This is how people start to pace themselves, convinced they will crash if they do 100 more steps. Do you notice this pattern? If you do, you are actually focused on danger, and not focused on the fact you can walk, so the protective brain will keep doing high arousal or shut you down.

You are better not doing an activity if you perceive it is dangerous, because you are making matters worse. You are exposing yourself to activity in a bad state, and like Pavlov's dogs, it will trigger the wrong physiology, reinforcing the survival response to triggers in future. Get focused before you do anything. Look for evidence that you can move and do not let a bad experience determine your future.

Focus on the fact that you are safe. Notice when you feel confident. A good way to do this is to recognise that if you aren't feeling concerned, then you must be feeling okay about it. Start by doing exercises that you know you can achieve; a few stretches and then shout out "I am OKAY!! I am safe; my body works! Build up your confidence. In the online *Reset to Thrive* training, there are great examples to prove to you that what you focus on is what you get; when you (or rather your chimp) is focused on danger, you can find it in everything, and you will be missing signs that the body can work. When we focus on what we can do, we start to find evidence everywhere.

You were hijacked by the lowered threshold, by the unconscious brain making connections, by the over vigilant meerkat and the overactive chimp or reptile, but now you can show them that you don't need them by focusing on your successes instead. When your body feels able, climb one step only and notice you did it! Start with something you *can* achieve then build on it.

If you are gung-ho, use your body whenever it feels okay and focus on what you can do. Even if you then need to rest or sleep for days, focus on what you did achieve. You will recover because you focus on the green, healthy track, noticing you are safe. You stop telling the protective brain that you are in trouble and need its assistance. Remember the body adapts, depending on whether you are safe or in danger.

5. Focus on what you have done, especially when you have crashed.
When you have a setback or not feeling good, think of all of moments when the body was working, and the protective brain was not running. Notice this when you lie in bed, or anytime the body feels relaxed. If you are able, write it all down. I have never met a person who didn't have evidence that their body works; if you are ever awake, able to move, or relaxed, it is working then.

When I used to crash (which was often!), I learnt to lie in bed, immobilised, sometimes for days, but I recited all the things I had done. "I did go to the shops! I *did* make a cup of tea! I *did* walk the dog a short distance; I *did* stay up for 6 hours. I *can*, I *will* and I'm *going to* again."

Focusing on the ups is essential for recovery. Make the brain focus on success, even if you have had to rest up again. From now on, everything is okay. You are going to consciously make the unconscious part of the brain recognise you are okay, that you don't need protecting. When you see the world as a safe place, you will turn off the malfunctioning survival system that has been creating mayhem. Even though you have symptoms, you are okay, you are going to get through this. Focus on being OKAY. Everything is OKAY.

EXERCISE: Focus on your recovery by keeping a journal every day. Notice when you are in the green track, your healthy parasympathetic system, with that lovely, juicy vagal system feeding every part of your body. Look for green shoots of recovery, any sign of success. Never discount the small stuff.

Keep a journal of successes to make yourself focus on what you want. Write down every tiny thing that tells you that you are better than at your worst, that there is an improvement. Record every moment when your body has not completely shut down or does not feel wired and in pain. Any time it feels better and can function.

These successes can be as small as noticing you managed to make a cup of tea or managed to get to the toilet on your own without crawling or holding onto the wall. Even if you crawled, as I did in the beginning, your body had some energy! Maybe you got downstairs, even if you couldn't get back up without resting. I could often be found at the bottom of the stairs asleep. Latch onto evidence of improvement with joy and gradually the body calms; a snowball effect is created. My body slept for days at a time, but when I came round, I focused on the fact that sleeping is a good thing, and that my body needed it. From little acorns, great oak trees grow. They are your seeds of recovery.

It is fantastic that you notice the big stuff as well, of course! You may notice that you were awake and able to do things for a few hours; that's amazing! Your body is running the healthy system. When your body is calm, that is evidence of recovery, as the chimp is resting.

If you remember better with pictures, take photos and videos or draw good moments. You could print off the photos or upload them onto a social media platform to have evidence of your focusing skills and evidence of a healthy moment. You can do audio recordings so you can go back and listen to it, especially in those times when you are not so good. Any smart phone or laptop today will have a recording facility.

These are statements from people who keep Recovery Journals. Write anything, everything, no matter how small, that tells you your body is working. Write it down and read it anytime you have a setback or need to remind yourself that you are on track. I have attached some examples below:

> *"As I lie in bed, my body is calm."* (*it is running in the healthy track!*)

> *"My body feels calm and relaxed watching television."* (*hurrah!*)

> *"I was able to get downstairs this morning, and I made a cup of tea standing up and felt fine."* (*Hurrah!!*)

> *"I read my book sitting up in bed for 30 minutes and felt OKAY."* (*My body can work!!*)

> *"I went for a 5-minute walk and felt good."* (*so happy!*)

> *"I made my bed and got dressed and I felt good!"* (*my body IS working- exciting*)

> *"I did 10 minutes of meditation when I woke up and felt*

really good." (Amazing!)

"I did 10 minutes of breathing exercises and focused; felt good afterwards for over an hour!" (so happy my body remembers what to do again)

"I noticed that I was able to keep going all morning, then rested and felt good again in the afternoon. (A big tick in the box)

"I went for a walk on the beach and I didn't crash afterwards." (walking is safe!)

"I got downstairs and then needed a rest at the bottom but I did it! (Hurrah!)

"I was able to sit up and hold my teacup and my body felt okay!" (Amazing.)

*" I walked for over a mile and felt good, **and** I didn't crash when I got home!" (I'm recovering!!!!)*

"I saw friends for coffee and was able to keep going; my body felt calm and was working!!" (BIG STAR)

"I have been feeling good all day today, did normal stuff; put bins out, cleared up, went for a walk, read emails, spoke to my sister for 10 minutes on the phone and made dinner". (Fantastic, so pleased)

"I walked around the block then crashed at the table, into my soup. BUT I DID IT!! (ecstatic!)

Of course, the people who wrote their journals had setbacks, but the exercise to shift focus is to train ourselves to look for signs of recovery; to look for what we want and what is useful for recovery.

People who keep up with journals get more rapid progress. Mick, the mountain bike champion, wrote down every tiny piece of evidence. As a mountain biker, he was brilliant at being focused, but the shock of being immobilised had terrified him; he went off track and had become brilliant at focusing on danger. To recover, he shifted his focus back to having a healthy focus, and noticing when he is safe. Focus on its own isn't enough but it is essential.

Obviously, the body hasn't fully recovered yet because this is the start of your journey, but when you notice it is working, you focus on being healthy and the body starts to revert to normal healthy mode.

Margaret's Story

Margaret couldn't walk unaided and had to be helped with everything, including drinking and feeding because she was so weak. On the first day of training, she noticed she could sit up on her own, and she was able to hold a teacup instead of having to have someone hold it for her. She wrote three pages of A4 notes on the tiniest things that told her that her body did have energy - it takes energy to be awake, to sit up, to write, and it takes energy to hold a cup. She carried on her journal every day for months, and it was a significant component in her recovery. Her brain started to register that she did have energy, that she was okay doing everyday tasks, safe, and it turned off the malfunctioning protective brain. She changed the way her body adapted to situations by getting it to recognise health, instead of always focusing on the illness and threats.

Be more like Margaret! The more it registers that you are healthy, the quicker your adaptive system switches off the protective system and returns to normal, permanently. That old mammalian system is only meant for life-threatening situations. It is not your fault that the brain is massively geared towards noticing danger; we are still more animal than human in evolutionary terms, so it is easy to get hijacked by the protective system. However, you need to consciously make the brain focus on health and make it get the message that you are safe.

F.E.E.D.

Neuroscientists appreciate that to switch from the protective systems to the thrive system, we need to focus, but we also have to put in the effort until it is effortless and be determined to keep it up. The acronym they use for this is F.E.E.D.

- Focus
- Effort
- Effortless
- Determined

Getting into F for Focus. A great nonverbal signal (NVS) for focus is the "blinkered horse" gesture. Horses are blinkered to make them focus and not get distracted by anything that isn't useful. Close your eyes, have your hands in front of you, fingers together, and place them at each side of your face, touching your temples. You may do this naturally when you want to concentrate. Anytime you need to focus, use this gesture to get you focused. There is another gesture; the single-handed gesture, which involves putting a straight hand up to your nose and directing it slowly forward, like an arrow focused on the target. You will see sports people use these gestures because they need to be focused in order to achieve.

The first E in F.E.E.D is for Effort. To establish new habits, we need to be aware of the old habits, consciously decide to stop them and to do something else until that becomes a habit. In the beginning you do have to make a conscious effort to look for signs of recovery and look for when you are functioning in the healthy track.

This does not mean that you are going to push through when you are feeling ill. This book is not about pushing through; there are no medals for forcing yourself to do something when the body is in the wrong physiology (when the healthy green track is turned off). You wouldn't keep going with the flu, so why would you think of doing anything if you are not feeling well? When neuroscientists argue for us to put in the effort and do the work, they mean that you will do things when the body feels it can do something, and then you will consciously notice that it is working for you. You will put in the effort to focus on the right things and put in the effort to master the FEARLESS resources. Writing your journal of successes is a good example of conscious effort.

The other E in F.E.E.D is for Effortless. When you have spent enough time practising the healthy habits in FEARLESS, one day you will notice that you do them automatically. One day, you get up and get on with life and don't even think about your body. This is the point that neuroscientists say it has become effortless, running for you unconsciously and automatically. Remember, when you follow in the footsteps of others who recover, you will be back to normal and taking it all for granted again; you will be out walking and living again. You will be in autopilot, focused on life, not your body. Hurrah!

D is for Determined. As Winston Churchill said, "Never, never, never give up". Who succeeds? The one who gives up or the one who is determined to keep doing what they need to do to achieve? I know that you are going to be determined to keep going because you bought a book on recovery! You will become brilliant at focusing on all the times (minutes or hours) that you are feeling healthy. Determination is not about pushing through when you feel awful or when your body is shutting down. Determination is the ability to stay on track and get back on track, even when you have setbacks, to achieve your goal. You will take time out if your body has had enough and stay calm, accepting that this is a normal part of recovery.

Exercise: Make a poster for your wall for the acronym F.E.E.D.

- Focus. Concentrate on any successes or signs of recovery that your body can work.
- Effort. Keep doing manageable small activities and consciously notice the evidence that your body is okay.
- Effortless. Keep it up until you notice the body is working automatically and you are FEARLESS again. Your body is working in autopilot again.
- Determined. Be determined to keep going, get back on track, and stay focused on the right stuff.

The E in FEARLESS is for
Excited, Ecstatic, Emotions

You can't be cautious and excited at the same time. We are going to stop being cautious because caution keeps defence mechanisms activated, and we are going to consciously activate healthy responses, that fire off the healthy systems, and let you thrive. When we are joyful, we fire off endorphins, which are the greatest healing molecules in the body and a proven pain killer. If you want to recover and reduce pain, fire off your endorphins. Stress chemicals increase pain and endorphins reduce pain. They are the most extraordinary chemicals, and we have them in our bodies! We just have to use them by turning them on. Shaking, laughter, rubbing and chanting all fire off the endorphins. This is why you feel good after a massage. So, celebrate, cheer! Fire off the healing chemistry and activate the healthy green track again. Reset to Thrive.

I remember being ecstatic that I had walked around the block and announced it with glee to my daughter as I entered the house. Ten minutes later I collapsed while having some soup. But I did it! I grinned in bed at my success. Celebrate your successes.

Like the excitement of finding tiny green shoots in springtime, you are going to be as excited about finding green shoots of recovery. This is why the healthy track is represented in green on your autonomic, adaptive diagram (ANS). You are looking for any evidence that it is working. Sadly, many people think they shouldn't get excited until they know they have no more symptoms. It is impossible to recover when you see everything as a problem and are focused on still having symptoms. When you magnify the danger, the protective system will stay on. And if you miss the evidence that sometimes you are okay, or dismiss it as unimportant, the malfunctioning chimp and reptile will keep you stuck.

Notice the difference between these two sentences:

- "I walked for 30 minutes today but my toe hurt when I got home". Already you feel defeated or are just trying to prove how poorly you are.

Now say it properly:

- "I walked for 30 minutes today! Fantastic, amazing, my body's working! I can recover, I already have evidence! It's okay if I have a sore toe at the end of it or need to rest for a while."

Celebrate to send the message home that you are okay. Every time you do the smallest thing, give yourself a pat on the back, shout out, "I DID IT!", punch the air, just anything that means something to you. As you walk, be excited, and celebrate every step. The brain will make healthy connections, and it will associate mobilising with safety, and reset from survival mode back to thrive mode.

Whenever you break into a smile or make joyous sounds, you are showing you are safe and so will automatically stimulate the healthy vagus nerve. You are back in control.

When you reward yourself with a "Well done" or a cup of tea, you fire off a chemical in your brain called dopamine that accelerates learning. Your amygdala will quickly learn that you are safe and capable, so recovery is much more rapid. Biologically, your brain needs rewards, so mark every good moment. Jill Bolte Taylor, a neuroscientist, describes her recovery from a stroke in *My Stroke of Insight* (2008). She emphasises that focus, and rewards are crucial for recovery; she celebrated everything, no matter how small. Her mantra was, celebrate every improvement. As a neuroanatomist, she knew how important it was to literally engrave every useful moment in the brain. If you are out of the habit of rewarding yourself, then just be fascinated that you do this, and commit to practising healthy habits that reset to thrive. No doubt this illness will have affected your self-esteem and identity, so it is essential that you are proud of yourself and your successes.

If you notice that you struggle with finding evidence or you dismiss it, then be amazed how brilliant you have become at focusing on the illness and getting stuck. It means your protective brain has been in charge for a long time, magnifying anything that could be dangerous. This is a Battle of the Brains, and your brilliant higher self is going to take control and break free from the chimp and reptile systems. The alternative is being a slave to the dominant protective brain. Be grateful for every sign of recovery. To reset to the thrive system, you need evidence that you are thriving.

The A in FEARLESS is for Adapt

When the environment is healthy, the body automatically resets to the parasympathetic nervous system (the thrive position). As Naviaux (2020, p41) said, healing and recovery only happens at a cellular level when organisms get the "all clear" signal that it is safe again. This is essential for recovery. You are going to make your world feel safe again. When you feel well enough to do anything, you will be excited. If you notice that you are very cautious, then it is good to start small and find ways to build your confidence. Do the Traffic Lights procedure: stop, engage in clear thinking, know you are safe, and find your courage and confidence to do just one step. You can do this.

Getting your confidence back is a huge part of recovery. Everything in your recovery pack is about working the healthy pathways; gradually getting back to normality and taking it for granted you can walk and do whatever you like. Confidence is the opposite of being fearful or wary. Remember, the whole point of this journey is to turn off the malfunctioning overprotective brain and turn the healthy system back on, permanently. You already have evidence that the healthy systems are functioning, intermittently. The journal, *Focusing on Recovery*, enables you to build your confidence and stop being fearful or anticipate disaster. It isn't normal to live in fear and it isn't healthy; you will just get evidence that your body is reacting badly to daily life. You are either thriving or surviving. Check out that you are feeling at ease when you do anything. Even when I was bedridden and unable to move, I consciously defied the protective brain and stayed calm, knowing, "this will pass, I'm okay, I'm safe and I don't need you".

Imagine you are the zookeeper, keeping the protective animals in our brain under control. The amygdala is hypervigilant, like a meerkat. Then we have the highly aroused chimp, trying to pump you up for any potential threats, and the ancient immobilising reptile, shutting down the body. You need to tame them and take control. Turn it into a game; it's you against the animal brain, and you are going to win and take control. The brilliant you, the higher human self, is not going to let some ancient relic of a survival brain run amok. You are going to do things within your remit and get evidence that you can; then the animal brain calms down. Start with anything you know you can do and then add on to it; just literally add one step at a time. All events and activities will then disconnect from the survival system and reconnect to the healthy system, letting you do things normally again.

Jill's Story

Jill had been ill for ten years and was achieving 50 steps a day outside. She couldn't get beyond 50 steps because she "knew she would crash". As Jill got closer to 50 steps, she anticipated disaster. Her body prepared for disaster, switching to the red track, and she felt dreadful. After doing 50 steps, she went indoors for the rest of the day. I suggested 50 was a conveniently round number; why did the body not stop at 49 or do 51? I asked what would happen if she did one more step, and she was horrified. When asked what would happen if she did one inch more, she replied, "that would probably be okay". I asked what would happen if she took 50 tiny steps - could she then do more steps, since she won't have gone as far as usual? It made no sense that the body would crash at 51 steps if she had only covered half the ground. By this time, we were laughing because we both appreciated that it didn't make sense! Many years before, she had bad experiences, and regularly crashed after "doing too much". She was then advised by specialists that she had to accept her condition, and that she was making herself worse by doing too much. They told her that the way to stop crashing was to do much less. So, she did.

I asked her to imagine that she had been put in a cage that only allowed her to pace 50 steps, but now she was going to break free! The "animals" had been keeping her in a cage; instead of her controlling them, they were controlling her. Every time she broke free, she was going to tell them, "See. I'm free; I don't need you!" and laugh. It is extraordinary, once you break free, how far you can go. Honestly, this lady was then able to walk 100s of paces and then walking became unlimited, as recovery progressed.

EXERCISE. This exercise allows you to break out of the limitations that were restricting you! Take just one extra step more than normal and break free from your cage. Take another because it is fun! If you think you can only do 50, do 51 with joy. Be childlike and free and take yourself back to a time in your life when you were free and feel what it feels like to do it like this.

I started by walking to the end of my short driveway (about five metres). Then, when I practised that and felt confident, I walked to the first lamppost. When I knew I could do that several times easily, I walked to the second and third lamppost. In between, I had many times when the body didn't work, which is to be expected initially, but focusing on success means the brain is relearning that the world is safe to explore. Mick, the mountain biker, measured paces around his house, then the garden, until he knew he could walk the same distance around the block. This way, you always know you are safe and can be confident.

If you go outside fearful then, of course, you take the chimp and reptile with you, and you will experience symptoms or crash. So please, when you go out, leave the chimp and the reptile in their box and go out excited, confident, and determined. Confidence is trusting yourself and trusting your body. You will trust your body when you start small and achieve. When the body has setbacks, be confident that this is normal in recovery.

Again, check out your nonverbal signals as I can't emphasise enough how they impact on the chimp, your vagal system and physiology. Is every part of you displaying confidence as you approach something? Any whisper of doubt is like a drop of arsenic in a glass of wine. Practise indoors; if you can do 300 steps indoors, logically you can then do them outdoors. You reset to thrive when you stop needing protection.

Make activities safe again by doing small manageable chunks, building up, and knowing they are safe. You were automatically conditioned to be protected, but you are now consciously reconditioning yourself to thrive. Be really proud of yourself.

R in FEARLESS is for Resilience and Rational

What else do we need to have on our journey to recovery? Resilience is needed because we have to pick ourselves up and start all over again when there are setbacks. Resilience takes courage and determination.

Resilience is an essential tool for life, so we will practise it now.

If resilience were an object, what would it be? For me, it is a bouncy blue ball because it keeps bouncing back. It's also one of the greatest gifts we can give to children. Life has ups and downs, but resilience means you never give up; when you are at the bottom, the only way is up. Children who are taught to get back up after a fall, or to try again, are the ones who will bounce back in adulthood. Resilience is the opposite of "marshmallowing", which is when you need to be wrapped in cotton wool; you stop doing anything that could be scary and limit your life to be safe. Marshmallowing gets you stuck. CFS associations, and sometimes our loved ones, marshmallow us out of kindness, but it is not useful. Needing to be safe means the survival brain is running the show.

Find one moment in your life when you were resilient - it doesn't have to be a big moment, but recall this moment, and remind yourself what it is to be resilient and how it made you feel proud. It could be when you fell off your bike and got back on, or when you went through a break-up, but you bounced back from it. One moment when you did manage to do something when you were ill. Challenges test our strength, but you can bounce back; you will recover when you choose to keep going, in the moments your body is in the green track. Call on your inner strength. Later, you will learn a technique to quickly access resilience and other healthy states needed for recovery.

Being rational is clearly a higher brain strategy; remember that the way to turn off your defence modes is to turn on your higher conscious brain. When you are rational, you will approach a problem calmly and clear headed, deciding how best to deal with it. If you notice that you are struggling with stairs or symptoms, you will stop any initial reactions from the chimp or reptile. Just take a deep breath to reset and give time to engage rational thinking, telling the chimp or reptile you are safe, and then when the body settles, you can proceed, just doing one step at a time. One step shows you can mobilise safely.

Get into the habit of saying "stop" anytime you notice inappropriate responses and engage your conscious brain. You know why this is happening. Stay calm - you do not need protecting. Role model the case studies mentioned and decide to deal with events and symptoms calmly and rationally. Everything is about turning off unconscious responses that you had no control over by becoming conscious and deciding how you want to respond instead. By doing this, you override the chimp and the reptile. Use the example of resetting yourself after a lorry has passed and you are safe, or any moment when you stop instinctive responses with rational thinking.

All the times when you weren't being hijacked by the chimp, you were rational. When you are resilient, your face is determined and in control, and you're facing the world, ready to try again. Your body is settled and strong, and your tone of voice sounds determined and in control.

L in FEARLESS is for Looking after Yourself

In my experience, many people with CFS have a difficult time really looking after themselves; they don't value their own health as much as they value others. To thrive, you must learn to care for yourself. If you were raised with Christian values, the commandment to remember is, "Love Thy Neighbour as Yourself".

Caring for yourself is not the same as marshmallowing. It is healthy to feel compassion for that person who is suffering (you) and what you are going through without doing the "woe is me" routine. It is healthy to tell yourself that you have had a tough time, as you would to others. Compassion is the antithesis of self-loathing, hostility, blame or frustration; compassion heals the body. David Hamilton, a pharmaceutical researcher turned healing speaker, clarifies what is happening chemically when we are unkind and self-loathing to ourselves, compared to when we are self-assured, compassionate, and fearless. The heart is affected by hostility, but the body heals itself when compassion fires off the "love drug" oxytocin. If you notice that you haven't been firing it off because you put yourself down, berate or devalue yourself, then this is an excellent time to start being compassionate. Likewise, feeling hostile to others isn't useful for recovery. Fill yourself with oxytocin as you begin to be kind and loving to yourself. In everything you do, do it with kindness for yourself. Know that every part of your brain is trying to do its best for you, and it always wants to look after you, stopping you in your tracks, if it detects you are struggling.

Whenever you notice the body is packing in, or you're feeling wired or in pain, instead of being frustrated with your body and yourself, be grateful that you have a brain that is doing its very best to protect you. Once you tell the chimp brain, very gently but firmly, that you don't need protecting, it will be relieved and relax. Would you be angry with a child or a friend for being unwell, or do you comfort them and reassure them? Wouldn't you take the pressure off them and say that getting better is more important than anything else at this moment? It is imperative that you work with yourself not against yourself: everything needs to be going in the same direction toward recovery. Every moment of every day, nurture compassion and be kind to yourself. If your body packs in, that's okay; you haven't done anything wrong. If your body is aching or heavy, stop. You are horrified by animal cruelty when a donkey is on its knees. So don't be cruel to yourself.

When you truly care for yourself, healing oxytocin flows through you, and leaves a lovely warm feeling inside. Practise saying "how clever are you" when you notice you did well today, or smile or laugh. Compassion is love and caring for yourself. It is not arrogance or pride, and it is not a sin. It is an essential part of health, recovery and well-being. The chimp will know it isn't needed when it notices you can look after yourself. So when you are lying in bed, give yourself a hug and be at peace; you will recover much quicker when you fire off the healthy hormones and the healing parasympathetic system. I spent a lot of time in bed just hugging myself. There wasn't a lot else to do, and I promise you it is infinitely better than berating yourself or being terrified, because that will just make you more ill. Oxytocin is the bonding chemical for attachment and one of the saboteurs to recovery is isolation, strife and hostility. If you are isolated, endeavour to have someone who can just be present, whether it's a buddy, a volunteer, or a pet. You will learn later just how important friendly social interaction is for health and well-being.

The second E in FEARLESS is for Emotional Detachment from a Threat

It is not enough to do a ten-minute mindfulness exercise or meditation and then revert to survival mode for the rest of the day. You will notice very little change doing that. You need to start living mindfully and noticing everything as an unaffected, curious observer. When you are detached and curious, you cannot be in survival mode.

Mindfulness enables us to wake up and become consciously aware, which allows us to access higher brain states. When you become mindful, the unconscious, mindless survival brain is inhibited. Mindfulness is simply to notice objectively without emotion, putting distance and space between you and the unhelpful event, then letting it pass. Just notice how you are feeling and responding to different triggers or moving. Notice sensations. Don't buy into fear or drama, but rather simply be curious and fascinated. Consciously return to the calm healthy system.

When you notice symptoms or are unable to move, every part of you, including your facial expression and auditory tone of voice must be calm and confident. Practise saying "It's okay" with a deep, reassuring tone, and take a breath from your diaphragm and relax. Everything will pass. If you are feeling highly aroused, with your heart beating through your chest, simply notice it, and watch it all going on from a distance. You are going to be a Mindful Observer, looking on, as you notice those flight and flight chemicals fly through your body.

EXERCISE: Close your eyes and notice how it feels to have space between you and the symptoms. You are observing them, not attached to them. Rise above the symptoms and as you feel separate from them, feel how safe you are. Notice that they are simply sensations and imagine them as something harmless or funny. You have become wise and knowledgeable, like a little Buddha. You understand what is happening and simply say, "it is okay, it will pass." You can take all of those sensations and put them on a train and watch them pass into the distance or let them float off in a hot air balloon. Smile and raise your face to the sky and be grateful. When you open your eyes, you will feel better and know you have reset your body. The symptoms may not have passed yet, but you have stopped firing off any more survival chemicals that had been creating the symptoms, so just let the chemicals dissipate. This can take a while, so it is a good idea to refocus on anything other than your body. Get utterly absorbed in something else while the chemicals dissolve and disappear. Notice your body language as you embody this calm, proud, patient Buddha figure, rising above everything and feeling at ease.

The First S in FEARLESS is for Serenity

"Give me the courage, to change the things I can,

The serenity to accept the things I can't,

And the wisdom to know the difference."

- The Serenity Prayer

These wise words are the essence of recovery. Wisdom is engaging your higher brain and developing knowledge, so that you will become better at knowing when to rest and when to get back to normal. It is learning to engage all the FEARLESS tools you are learning about.

Accept when the body needs a rest and know when to have courage to keep going, no matter how many setbacks you encounter. You will become better at listening to your body and better at using the tools. It is okay to err, that's part of improving. If you have seen experts or been involved in CFS support groups and associations, there is a good chance you have started accepting the condition and do adaptive pacing. We are not talking here about accepting the condition, we are talking about the moments when your body needs to rest or when you have symptoms and need to let them pass. Then, you are going to calmly try again.

Serenity is so essential. When you lie in bed immobilised, develop a deep sense of calm. There is nothing wrong with your body; it is simply ticking over like a stationary car; be assured *there is no damage,* even if your metabolism has gone out of synch whilst in survival mode. Be at peace, accepting that the body will stay in protective mode until it is safe to mobilise. As you rest, give all your worries to the universe or whatever you want to give it up to. Send it off and let it go; you will feel so much lighter.

When I lay in bed, terrified, I used to say: "I am too small to deal with this myself, so I am giving this problem over to a higher power, and as I let go of all concerns, I am simply going to do what I can do: rest easy, and wait for this to pass." Release the burden and feel peace. Turn terror into serenity; it is your primary tool. I promise you, the act of letting go, and giving it to something greater than yourself and waiting serenely for it to pass, will provide you with peace.

When you have weird, extraordinary symptoms caused by the red track, your heart may be racing, and you may feel wired, nauseous and in pain. You may have acute sensitivity to light, so that any light feels like a laser piercing through your eyes, or you may have such hypersensitivity to noise that any sound creates pain in your ears. Whatever your symptoms are, the fact is you have been thrown into a primal state of heightened arousal, and you need to let it settle. Hang on in there, just notice the sensations from a detached distance, and be patient. Everything will pass when you let it. You don't know when, but it will. Any fear will heighten the pain and symptoms, making you more ill.

Serenity will come when you truly believe you will recover and keep the faith. It is a choice to have faith in the future and to trust you will be okay. Choose to have faith in the future and trust you will be okay. Even in your darkest moments, focus on the rainbow to give you peace. Your body needs restfulness to heal.

In the early days of CFS, when I was mostly asleep and desperate, I wrote poetry to let go of my negative emotions. Do anything that helps you keep perspective and stay serene, have faith, and find your courage. It is okay to feel momentary despair, but it is not okay to hold onto it. Let it go by writing, or screaming in a wide-open field, or crying, and then let it pass. I had a rule that after twenty minutes of being emotional, I had to stop, take a breath, refocus, and believe again that I would recover. You will get over this. Believe, stay calm, and keep your courage.

And pack a load of humility and amazing grace on your journey because this illness makes us humble. It teaches us that we are not Superwoman or Superman, and it exposes us as "weak" when we desperately want to be strong and be seen as strong. To learn humility is to learn that it is okay to have weaknesses because we are human. We are not God.

What does serenity feel like for you? How is your face, body and tone of voice as you are gently, compassionately accepting? You will feel at ease, soft and light. When have you ever felt at peace, serene and accepting? Find one moment and practise these healthy resources.

The Second S in FEARLESS is for Seeing Things Differently

Like all organisms, when you perceive your surroundings to be healthy, your body will adjust accordingly. Clearly, changing our perception is a conscious decision and requires us to be rational. Once again, we are exercising the higher brain to override the malfunctioning survival systems which are causing the illness. I know so many people get stuck because they are terrified of symptoms, and hence keep their survival brain running. When you change your perception of events and symptoms, you literally change your physiology.

When the amygdala learns that activity is scary or too demanding, it puts you into survival mode. To retrain the amygdala, you need to perceive everything is safe so your body will run automatically in the healthy physiology. Changing perception is one of your greatest tools; it is a game-changer. There is no damage, no matter how weird and powerful the symptoms are. In arousal, it is just chemicals swishing around your body. With shutdown and crashing, it is your body ticking over, functioning but not moving. You are safe.

When I was bedridden initially, I had no idea what was happening, and the symptoms were terrifying; my body seemed to slosh around uncontrollably. Then I realised that the body was malfunctioning, sending out crazy loads of chemicals that were creating bizarre symptoms. Having that understanding meant symptoms were no longer scary. I decided just to be mindful, observing symptoms from a distance, but I also changed my perception of the event; I saw symptoms as funny or ridiculous sensations. I imagined them as a bathful of water, being swished around all directions. Everything passes when you let it and I knew I just had to ride out.

I became fascinated by all sensations. When you know what is happening, you do not need to be scared of crashes or any other symptoms. Become fascinated, curious, and calm. Symptoms are just sensations, so hang on in there until they pass. See them as something harmless and ridiculous. When you do it like this, you will notice rapid progress.

You cannot be fascinated by a sensation and terrified of it at the same time. So changing the perception of the event turns off the malfunctioning survival mechanisms and your body will revert to calm mode, re-adapting naturally to a safe world.

Jane's Story:

Jane was experiencing nausea and sickness symptoms all morning until we spoke. She was asked to change her language, from talking about symptoms to seeing them as sensations, because symptoms are associated with illness, and it isn't useful to focus on illness. I then asked her to imagine the sensations being like butterflies, fluttering around inside. (She had no fear of butterflies, so you need to choose something that is a pleasant sensation). She was then asked to do a mindfulness exercise, to observe the butterflies and detach herself from them. Then she needed to dissociate, by letting the butterflies get on with what they are doing while she focused on getting on with her life. This is where focus is so important; she had to fill her mind with something other than the sensations. She became absorbed in transplanting seedlings. The brain doesn't register the sensations when it is 100% focused on something else. This gave the body time to allow the chemicals to dissipate without being triggered again. She contacted me to say that she felt good again.

There is no magic, except the magic of the brain and its mastery over the body. We change our perception of our world by seeing things differently, bigging up successes, focusing on those successes, and minimising threats, thereby taking the power away from symptoms. Notice in the Journal of Recovery examples how much we need to big up and magnify any successes and get everything into a healthy perspective again. When we focus on recovery, the brain perceives a healthy world and when we focus on problems, the brain perceives threat and the body adapts accordingly. The more you change your perception of symptoms, the more the brain registers that you are safe, and won't need to be rescued by the survival brain.

FEARLESS: Role Model Success

Here are wonderful examples to role model for recovery from Long Covid, PVFS and CFS:

"I want to say I am in week 14, 95 days. I AM getting better. I did a 25 min walk on Monday and drove to the beach yesterday for ice cream and a 10-minute walk (shorter to balance out the longer drive). Today I am tired but haven't totally crashed out. Laying on the sofa is fine. It feels both huge in progress, and also tiny at the same time. I cheer myself on, then laugh at how funny it is to be so proud of such a tiny thing, then cheer again!" - Nic, a Covid-19 sufferer and nurse, in recovery.

Note the language "I am tired but haven't totally crashed"; this is a person keeping things in perspective and while calmly, acknowledging tiredness, she is emphasising that she didn't crash. She is using all the right FEARLESS tools in her recovery pack; celebrating to mark the moment, cheering herself on. She is laughing and firing off endorphins that heal the body and she is doing it with compassion and love for herself. She is not beating herself up because she is tired or berating herself for having only managed a tiny bit of activity. Furthermore, she is building up her level of activity and doing everything fearlessly. I can't emphasise enough how important all these FEARLESS resources are for recovery. Fire off the healthy chemicals for every tiny success. Nic has an excellent approach, so it is little wonder she is recovering from Long Covid. Look at your checklist for FEARLESS resources and just notice how many Nic is doing for each tiny activity. You can role model Nic and all the other people doing it the right way. Tick off how many FEARLESS resources you successfully use every day.

If you notice the body has had enough, I suggest you rest or relax on a sofa. Then try again. Be gentle on yourself. Symptoms recur on the road to recovery, so expect this to happen. Dr Paul Garner, an epidemiologist who contracted Coronavirus, relates recovery to that of Dengue, whereby symptoms can come back out of the blue for up to six months or more.

Use the serenity prayer and accept the things you cannot change and the courage to change the things you can. As you start to feel a bit better, you will begin to mobilise, taking it easy at first and pacing yourself fearlessly and sensibly. You will stop when your body has had enough and be completely okay about it. Make the most of it. If you can, read, watch fun programmes you love, and eat healthy food and treats. Everything about recovery is about remaining calm all the time, whether you have symptoms and when you feel better. If you feel too ill to eat, take Complan or an equivalent health food drink; I lived on them for months once I was able to get out of bed but couldn't stand up for long enough to make something healthy to eat.

If recovering from Long Covid or viruses, even though you are ill, imagine you are filling receptors in the immune system with happy hormones and anti-viral molecules; when they are full up, the virus has nowhere to lodge. You need to be feeding back that, "even though I have a virus, I am okay", using your facial expression, tone of voice and relaxed breathing to assist recovery.

When viruses recur after recovery, it takes courage and resilience to keep bouncing back. I know when I have become emotional about contracting a virus again, and terrified that this time, I am going to end up bedridden again, I get stuck. Of course I do, just as you will get stuck if you get emotional for too long. It is entirely natural but also a massive saboteur for recovery. Get reassurance from a nurse or GP; go to someone who reminds you that you will get over this. Then get out your bouncy ball, or whatever is your object for resilience, and grab a handful of courage, to bounce back and recover properly.

For grit, determination, and strength, I imagine a steel rod going all the way from my head to my toes, holding me up like a pillar of strength. Originally, I envisaged a sword going up and through my spine, with the handle keeping my shoulders upright and broad. It doesn't matter what you use but call on it whenever you need to summon your courage and strength again. Symbols are powerful because our brains are brilliant at understanding symbolic meaning; as you read this, your brain is recognising every letter as a symbol for a sound, to make words. Art is a visual symbol and musical notes symbolise sounds, so attach symbols to each resource in FEARLESS. Here is a true story of someone with grit and a fighting spirit:

> *"The mindset of having the Olympian Spirit pulled me through. Others were pulling their masks off their face, speaking to family, and ten minutes later, were carried out in a black bag. I had this mask on, and my mind went back to Mexico City when I had an oxygen mask on, training for the Olympics. I said to myself, 'If I'm going to win this race, then this is the preparation I need to pull me through'. There*

were two men on the ward, one 82-year-old and the other an 84-year-old. Both were determined to pull through. Every hour on the hour, 24 hours a day, they would get up, walk around the ward, up and down. I thought, 'if they are doing it, I have to do it'. I got up ...collapsed and tried again...I said to myself, 'If you don't use it, you lose it.'" - Kenny Dwan, Olympic Medallist, recovering from Covid-19. (Radio 2 interview. Jeremy Vine Show May 2020)

You don't need fight and flight, you just need to call on your fighting spirit. One's fighting spirit is not sufficient for everyone who had Covid, but it is essential for you now, if you have Long Covid fatigue or CFS. I say, "Come on, you can do this: get a grip." Laugh at yourself if you falter, saying, "What are you like!" Being terrified of staying ill or of being ill again is natural, but it isn't an option for recovery.

Consistency

It is pointless doing the vagal exercises in the next chapter if you then spend the rest of the day turning on the chimp and reptile modes. You cannot do a ten-minute yoga, breathing or mindfulness exercise, and then revert to shallow breathing and unhealthy patterns for the rest of the day, because that will just reactivate the malfunctioning system that is causing the illness. Try to think of it this way:

- Imagine a fence:
- The fencing is your ongoing daily life.
- The posts represent healthy exercises.

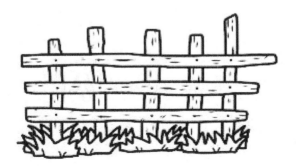

Doing your exercises or walking is great, but if you then spend the rest of the day avoiding triggers, focusing on symptoms or feeling anxious, your fence won't function properly. You need to have strong posts, doing activities intermittently, but crucially, you need to live your life the right way all the time, and doing it how you are meant to: mindfully, fearlessly, and using all the FEARLESS tools.

So many people with CFS think a massage or manicure is helpful, but then they revert to unhealthy patterns for the rest of the day. One step forward and ten steps back. Many CFS websites advocate having a manicure or massage to "feel better", but it is only a sticking plaster, and of little use for recovery. Massage fires off the healthy endorphins, so you will feel good initially, but it is temporary relief. In normal daily life, we see people doing this all the time. Instead of changing their lifestyle, they think they are doing something useful to redress their stress, by doing a half hour workout or going to the pub, but that is not sufficient.

Consistency is absolutely key to success. Consistently practise the things in your FEARLESS toolbox so that they become a way of life, and not simply an exercise.

Summary

You are going to:

- Increase the threshold back to the normal range by doing reasonable, achievable activity. The chimp and reptile will only kick in if demands are, or are perceived to be, too much.
- Make the world safe and manageable, so the body naturally switches back to thrive mode.
- When activity is safe, the healthy vagal system will run again, giving you recovery. Fear and anxiety about activities will keep you in survival mode.
- Engage the higher brain to override the lower survival instincts.
- Notice when you are in the healthy green track, parasympathetic track, functioning normally, even if only for moments initially.

You need to expose yourself to tasks and activities when you feel okay, and do bite-size pieces that are achievable, so they stop being automatic triggers affecting the body. Then the amygdala registers you are okay, and you reset to thrive mode. You haven't fully recovered yet, so of course you will still have some symptoms. You have lived life healthily before, so you can do it again, no matter how long you have been ill.

It is normal to turn off the survival mechanism. You will practise approaching everything using your healthy FEARLESS resources to activate the thrive mode again. Then the dysfunctioning chimp and the reptile are no longer needed.

EXERCISE: HEALTHY FEARLESS RESOURCES. Write down everything you are going to put in your recovery pack. Copy out this list and pin it up:

Focus on what you want and record your successes in a written journal or voice record. Notice when your body can and does work for you.

Excited. Be enthusiastic about your successes.

Adapt. Your body will function according to the environment it is in. Practise finding successes within your environment, whether it is doing stairs, or walking in and out of your house, one step at a time. Turn it into a game of escaping from the prison that the protective brain had put you in. Healthy surroundings equals a healthy body.

Resilience. Keep bouncing back. Whenever there are setbacks, muster up your courage and strength. Use your Traffic Lights procedure to stop any panic or unwanted reaction. Engage rational thinking and proceed in a better state.

Love and care for yourself fully. Get social and emotional support.

Emotional detachment and calm mindfulness. Be a fascinated observer.

Serenity, wisdom, and amazing grace.

See Things Differently. Change perception of all activity. Your amygdala is using the perception of events to determine safety or danger, and adjusts the body accordingly. Turn symptoms into harmless, funny sensations.

EXERCISE. For each of these healthy, FEARLESS resources, give it a symbol. I used a rubber ball for resilience and a strong fence for consistency. Also give the belief that you can recover its own symbol.

- Draw a picture of a travel bag with all the symbols inside or import images of the symbols from online. Label each one. You can have a bag with real objects if this is preferable.
- You can attach a piece of music to each resource, so a particular song or piece of music represents one aspect of FEARLESS. Something calm for serene and something exciting for excitement. Play them often and remind yourself what they represent for you.
- Consistently FEARLESS. Remember that these resources are part of life, not just a ten-minute exercise each morning.

We are **not** packing the saboteurs such as frustration, blame, or catastrophising. Why would you want to take them on your journey? Put them in another bag and stick them in a cupboard. Better still, throw them behind you into the ether. Put the chimp and the reptile back in their box and keep them there, unless there is real, life-threatening danger, and only then, can they pop up to look after you.

Chapter 5: The Road To Recovery, Part 2: Work The Body

If we don't fire off the healthy pathways in our body, we lose them. Healthy pathways should be running in autopilot, but when they aren't used, they become slow and difficult to get going. Stroke and heart patients need to rehabilitate as soon as possible after the event occurred, to get the healthy pathways working. Likewise, you need to use your body, just as much as you need to use all the FEARLESS resources associated with thriving. When we shake our body, dance, rub our skin, jump, and walk around, we automatically fire off the endorphins, which heal and relieve pain. It is good to move, so that your body resets and recovers. Moderate exercise releases chemicals to improve learning and memory, thus, helping alleviate the brain fog reported by patients.

I was so stunned by the CFS world, having come from a background of teaching health and recovery, because they caution against using your body, saying you will pay for it, and it's your fault if you crash. No one is saying to run a marathon, but you do have to use your body confidently, when it is in the thrive mode, and stop when it starts to tell you that it has had enough, then repeat. You will learn that when you do it like this, the body rehabilitates itself. As research shows: "HPA axis changes can be reversed by modifying behavioural features of the illness, such as inactivity, deconditioning and sleep disturbance" (Cleare, 2004 p.55). So, we will increase activity, break the conditioned hardwiring between triggers and our protective system and improve restorative sleep.

Before even considering walking, it is essential to activate your healthy vagal system, in the parasympathetic mode, represented as the green track in our diagram. As you will recall, it runs through your body, connecting your auditory system, facial expression and vocal cords to your lungs, heart, gut and immune system. It is the one that enables you to thrive, heal and repair.

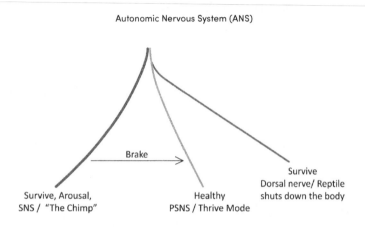

Autonomic Nervous System (ANS)

Brake

Survive, Arousal,
SNS / "The Chimp"

Healthy
PSNS / Thrive Mode

Survive
Dorsal nerve/ Reptile
shuts down the body

When survival modes are running, the healthy vagal system is compromised. You have already learnt to turn off the survival mode and reactivate the healthy system, by reacting with FEARLESS resources.

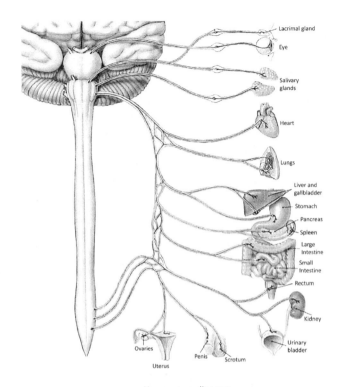

Vagus nerve diagram

Now, we can also reactivate the healthy systems, the green track, by using the parts of the body that are attached to the ventral vagus nerve in the healthy, relaxed parasympathetic system, our normal default mode.

Signs of low vagal tone, and of a deactivated vagal system, are fatigue, digestive problems, difficulty swallowing, brain fog, and shallow and flat muscle tone in the face. When it is deactivated during your illness, you may also notice bloated stomach, pain, inflammation of the joints such as with fibromyalgia, and rapid or slow bowel movements. Sound familiar?

There is no damage in your body; the healthy, vagal system turned off when the survival system turned on. Like an accelerator pedal and a brake pedal in a car, you can't use both at the same time. Now we need to do exercises to switch the vagus nerve back on, knowing it is appropriate to use the body again, assuming you have had plenty of rest after the virus or having initial crash. Weeks of complete restorative rest, initially, is essential to let the body heal; it is what other mammals do. Once the body feels up to it, and you want to move forward, there are many exercises you can do confidently, and which require minimal excursion.

We will start with vagal activation exercises and then look at how we use the body to get it back to normal functioning. If we look at the graph, the tolerance level has been reset with CFS, post viral fatigue syndrome (PVFS), or Long Covid, so the body goes beyond its tolerance level at the slightest effort or demand on it. You may feel as if you have peaked at 10% capacity, and then feel fatigue and ill health, as metabolisms and functions just tick over in survival mode.

Therefore, you need to start with small steps and build up the level of tolerance as the hypothalamus learns that it is safe to reset the threshold back to the normal, healthy level. Please note, the normal healthy level is not 100% capacity; healthy people function on about 85% capacity, leaving room to deal with unexpected burdens, infections, and viruses, or demands if they arise.

Diagram showing CFS / PVFS, Long Covid
has reset the body to a lower threshold

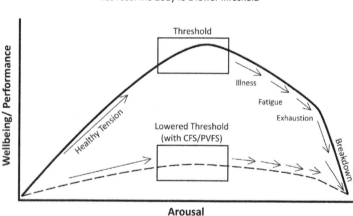

In the next chapter, we will learn a rapid technique to reset the body but for now, as you are building your confidence and strength, mastering the FEARLESS toolkit, it is a good idea to go gently and play with doing activities again.

It is essential to use your resourcefulness as you start to use the body. Whether you are singing, standing, sitting up or walking, you need to be doing them FEARLESSLY, You will endeavour to only expose yourself to exertion when you are using healthy resources and when your body feels able to do something. What fires together wires together, so do activities being healthy and safe.

FEARLESS stands for:

Focus on when you can do things.

Excited. Be enthusiastic, positive emotions.

Adapt. Make everything safe, doing bite-size manageable tasks.

Resilience. Be determined and courageous, bouncing back after setbacks. Stay calm and rational.

Love and care for yourself, fully. Get loving support.

Emotional Detachment and Mindfulness. Rise above fear and physical symptoms, an objective observer.

Serenity, courage, gratitude, and grace. Acceptance and letting go.

See Things Differently. Your amygdala is relying on perception, to know which track to send the body down. See triggers and symptoms as okay, then the body can reset. Nonverbal signals tell you if you are seeing things healthily. Smile, be uplifted and confident.

Vagal Activation Exercises

A simple acronym to remember how to activate your body is BETTER. Just as with FEARLESS, always have this acronym handy, to keep you on track. BETTER stands for:

Breathing exercises and meditation.

Exercise the body.

Throat exercises. Gargle, blow, sing, chant, to activate the vagus nerve.

Traffic Lights procedure to activate the higher, thinking brain and stop unhealthy habits.

Enjoy activity to thrive, only when the body feels up to it.

Rest peacefully and naturally, as anyone would when they have done a lot.

And you will have **BETTER** recovery, doing it this way. Get into the habit of doing these restorative meditations and breathing exercises. They are available online at www.resettothrive.co.uk

B in BETTER is for Breathing Exercises

Breathing exercises will stimulate the vagus when we breathe from our stomachs and use the diaphragm. Breathing from the chest sends a signal to the brain that you are in distress, and it fires off the SNS, turning off the healthy vagal activity. In an article to the National Journal of Physiology, Pharmacy and Pharmacology, Surekharani Chinagudi (2014) explains:

> *Various types of breathing exercises have various effects on the autonomic nervous system, like fast breathing increases sympathetic tone and slow breathing increases parasympathetic tone. Effect of slow deep breathing for a*

*short duration of five minutes in healthy adults who are not
practising any kind of breathing exercise or yoga is a shift of
the cardiac sympathovagal balance towards the sympathetic
predominance.*

If your body feels like this, it just means you haven't been using the body
properly for breathing. You are aiming to do five to seven breaths per
minute, but for now, focus on slowing your breathing. Start gently and
slowly build up. If you have been shallow breathing, now you need to
breathe naturally again. As well as stimulating the vagus nerve, needed
for healing and health, breathing also stimulates molecules of emotion,
which are called neuropeptides. One of these is endorphin, so breathing
exercises naturally alleviate pain. This explains why breathing exercises
are so effective in Hypnobirthing. Here are various breathing exercises
you can do, breathing in through your nose:

- Sit comfortably in a chair or your most comfortable place. Put a
  hand on your tummy and imagine you are blowing into a balloon
  in your tummy; notice your belly expands out gradually and
  easily. Take a slow deep breath in through your nose. Hold your
  breath for as long as is comfortable and feel at one with your
  body, connected to yourself. Now gently and deeply breathe
  out. Practise making the out breath longer than the in breath. If
  you are lying down, you can have a real or imaginary object on
  your tummy, and watch it rise to the ceiling as you inhale, then
  come back down as you exhale.
- Another breathing exercise using your diaphragm and pushing
  out your tummy, is known as four square breathing or Box
  Breathing; it is perfect for settling the sympathetic nervous
  system. Imagine sketching a square as you breathe - the first
  line is an in breath, the next an out breath, taking two cycles
  to complete the square. Inhale to a count of four and exhale to
  a count of four as you visualise your square. Breathe about a
  second per count then gradually with practise, make each count
  slower. 1234 will become 1...2...3...4...This exercise combines the
  vagal benefits of slow respiration and balanced breathing. Great
  for when we feel out of balance.
- Change the shape to a rectangle and repeat the exercise,

inhaling for the first short line, and exhaling for longer, on the long line, to activate vagal breathing. Visualise your rectangle as you breathe. With practise, slow the count.

- Practise blowing bubbles and feel what it feels like to blow a stream of bubbles! Such an easy exercise, and so joyful in working the body! Remember to push out your tummy when breathing.

- Buy a cheap instrument, a kazoo or a penny whistle, and blow. It doesn't matter what sound you make but remember to use your diaphragm and push your tummy out and in. If you can mobilise, go to open spaces, and make as much noise as you like.

- This next exercise is lovely to do outside or by an open window. Add music if preferred.

Sit or lie comfortably, with your eyes closed. Breathe deeply from your diaphragm, pushing your tummy in and out, for a count of three.

Feel the rhythm as you push your stomach out, to breathe in, and bring your tummy back in as you breathe out. Feel your body drawing in this beautiful air, filling you with life, and spreading through every part of your body. Give it a colour so you can see it spreading through you, nourishing you. Breathe out through your mouth for longer... gradually, over time, breathing out twice as much as you breathed in. Feel your body relax as you breathe out, noticing the tension fading. As you release carbon dioxide, consider how grateful the trees are to be drawing in your breath. Feel how much a part of the universe you are, and how we are all connected. Refocus on your body, breathing in and enjoy feeling what it feels like to be calm.

Draw energy back into your core, giving you inner strength. Feel what it feels like to retain your energy within. Let all the energy in your head spread down into your core, allowing your head to settle, all that exists is your breathing. Stay with this calmness for as long as you like, keeping the breathing in and out. Place your hands wherever is most comfortable and where your core energy rests. Then, when you feel ready, gradually move your head, take a deep breath in and breathe out deeply... open your eyes and feel your body recover.

It doesn't matter how long your body is calm, even a few seconds shows that you can do it. Use this exercise anytime you need to retrain the body to settle.

The E in BETTER is for Exercise.
Moving your body

The chimp turns on if supply can't meet demands, so you are only going to do things that are reasonable and when your body is in the right track to meet the demands. You cannot mobilise if the reptile or chimp tracks are activated. Exercise when supply can meet reasonable demands, doing everything with FEARLESS resources. Here are some examples:

- When you take a shower, do your breathing to prepare, then turn the temperature down to cool for a few seconds, either at the end or midway. You can decrease the temperature as your body adjusts to it. As you adapt to the cold, increase the time you have a cooler shower; you may gradually build up to 20 to 30 seconds, which is plenty for activating the vagus nerve. Go easy. When you recover, you can access the Wim Hoff technique on numerous free apps for deeper vagal activation exercises. www.wimhofmethod.com/instructors/catpaterson

- Swimming can also help you utilise your body and to help improve your breathing. The Total Immersion technique has specific, useful exercises on breathing, which you can access online or on DVD. Swimming is a particularly beneficial vagal exercise as you are using your body safely and breathing correctly. I find the Total Immersion method much more efficient and conserves energy, compared to traditional methods. It allows you to glide, flow and gently breathe.

- Do a little dance, shake, and twist, jump and skip, laugh. Never time yourself or set yourself limits as this implies you are going to "pay for it" if you do too much. In fact, you will crash if you are scared to dance, as the survival system will kick in. Remember when dancing was fun? Do a normal, healthy response.

- Walking stimulates the whole body. It doesn't matter if you are walking around your room or walking a hill; the body needs to move. You do not have to go far; you can walk in your house, in your garden or around the block. It is all about moving courageously and joyfully. Even if you can only do a few steps in your house, that's great; you will be amazed how many you can do. Then gradually build up. If you can do 50 steps inside the house, logically you can do 50 steps outside. If you have become programmed to shut down after 50 paces, stop counting and simply enjoy walking, initially around your house. Do what you know you can do easily and be joyful. Then gradually do a bit more, repeat over several days and then increase again.

- If you notice a tiny bit of fear creeping in, use the Traffic Lights procedure. Stop, decide if that is useful, take a breath, and recall all the times in life when you moved joyfully and confidently. Defy the meerkat, chimp, and reptile, be confident and once the body is settled, do one thing to prove you can mobilise!
- There are many free online yoga and meditation exercises online, so start with beginner courses and do what you can.
- If you are bedridden, check that this is the right time to mobilise. In bed, practise being FEARLESS by noticing when you can sit up, hold your head up, or sit on the edge of the bed. Sitting up on your own requires energy to move, so be proud of being able to do this. Do any exercise that gets the body working again. Then rejoice and mark the moment. You can do the breathing exercises in bed.

That's how I started. I managed to get to the toilet, initially by holding onto walls or crawling. Then one day, I managed to walk there and was ecstatic. Even crawling is good; it means you are not stuck in bed, and you are moving! Start to notice every movement you *can* do. Every movement is progress and will activate the vagus nerve, returning you to your healthy natural state. When you feel you can move more, build up your confidence and get successes.

T in BETTER is for Throat
Exercises to activate the vagus nerve

- **Gargle** to stimulate the ventral nerve in your throat and vocal cords. Each time you brush your teeth, gargle for about 20 seconds or do three ten second sessions a day, if the vagal nerve hasn't been stimulated in a while. Do this every day. Water is fine, but you can add your favourite mouthwash.

- Activate the vagus nerve in your throat and vocal cords by singing, chanting, or doing a celebratory whoopee. This turns on higher states of consciousness, thereby turning off the protective brain, and releases endorphins that are beneficial for your well-being. If you feel self-conscious, take yourself to a private place or a wide-open space and express yourself joyfully. Again, breathe from the tummy and use the diaphragm as you do vocal exercises. Express yourself, show up, be uplifted.
- Go to www.resettothrive to see how singing and breathing exercises are non-medical interventions to help people with COPD (chronic obstructive pulmonary disease) or any respiratory condition that causes long term breathlessness, including Long Covid. They have a free home exercises page and an advice sheet on managing fatigue after Covid-19 on their website www.thecheynegang.com
- Playing the kazoo or penny whistle will also activate the vagal system in the throat, as well as being a good breathing exercise.

The Additional T in BETTER is for the Traffic Lights Exercise

As our supply of energy increases, we can then increase demands, until we are back to the normal healthy threshold. If you are still being affected by basic activities, then this is a crucial time to stop and reactivate the healthy vagal system. Protective patterns are powerful and automatic; instinct and conditioned responses are unconscious, and it is how the brain naturally functions.

This is the Pavlovian response, or classical conditioning we discussed in the science chapter. Something, such as stairs or tasks, will trigger a response in your body. You have unwittingly become conditioned to shut down for things that used to be neutral events. What fires together, wires together. It is not anyone's fault, and we can override it with conscious discipline.

Remember your threshold level has been reset to shut you down for the slightest effort, as a protective mechanism. Anyone who has been bedridden because of an illness, needs to gradually build up their strength, but with CFS, we are also battling the protective reptile, which literally cuts the circuit and makes us crash. The illness is not that you are physically out of conditioning and need to get fit, but that your body has been shut down and is just ticking over. It is a terrifying experience; no wonder protection became the default mode. Such trauma is meant to prevent you from going near activity in the future, just as a horse-riding accident may put you off riding again. Whilst it is a perfectly normal protective response, it is not useful, and it will not help you to recover.

This is back to a Battle of the Brains. You need to become conscious of the pattern, engage the human brain and respond how you want to. You became a victim of the protective brain, but now you can take control and be in charge again. Be excited about being empowered again, choosing how your body responds!

Becoming Aware

Notice what makes you feel cautious, anticipate disaster, or have physical symptoms. Triggers could be physical load: stairs, hills, distance, paces or enforced activity. They may be social and emotional triggers, such as having to deal with social challenges, or they could be mental overload, being asked a question or making decisions.

The brain attaches meaning to time and distance; you are fine for 10 minutes, but then, if you go over 10 minutes, the amygdala switches on the chimp and reptile, detecting that the demand is too much. You may be able to do 50 paces in a healthy state but feel dreadful at 51 steps. It knows you are safe up to fifty steps, so you stay in the calm branch, but as you approach your fifty paces, the sympathetic is activated because a threat is detected. In life, survival mode switches on if you are about to walk off a cliff, but doing one extra pace is *not* life threatening, so we need to break that hardwiring. Conditioning is a quick, efficient way for the brain to learn because it is effortless, instant and requires no energy. However, it doesn't always develop healthy connections, especially when you had bad experiences, so become aware of what triggers inappropriate reactions in your body.

What to do, when you notice you are physically affected by triggers?

Changing Your Automatic Response: Start to become aware of how you respond to triggers. How does your body react? Do you crash, feel physically wired, become fearful, avoid doing things? Have you learnt that you must limit activity? Are you focused on pay back?

Write down your thoughts, what you hear yourself saying and doing. The reward for avoiding or limiting activity is to feel safe in your limited life. But you want more! You want to thrive again. You need to be aware of the stimulus causing your reactions, and then consciously change your response, not avoid the triggers.

This is a message I received from a lady who is successfully recovering from Long Covid symptoms:

> *"Perhaps your post Jan and what you describe about calmness and gentle movement explains what happened when I was out walking in the woods, feeling like wading through treacle, not being able to walk very fast, and being worried about having to walk uphill back to the car. When I just ambled along, resigned to the fact that I could only go very slowly and that it would take me ages but that it didn't matter, SUDDENLY the treacle feeling lifted, something cleared from my body, and my legs felt light and normal again. I walked at a normal pace and walked uphill without a second thought! It was such a definite lifting of something oppressive that stopped my body from functioning properly, so maybe, what you say about the Autonomic Nervous System malfunctioning is the reason?! Thank you so much for your words, they give me hope. "- Kristin, Long Covid Recoveree.*

This lady noticed her body felt like it was wading through treacle and her initial response to the trigger, the hill, was to be worried about walking uphill to get back to her car. This response would then usually cause her body to get worse and stop her in her tracks. So, she changed her perception of the trigger, and she changed her response.

Her new response was "everything is fine and safe", and suddenly her body went back to working normally. It isn't magic; by changing her response, she was able to proceed. She did STOP - THINK - GO. She switched off the overprotective brain and turned the healthy, calm physiology back on. Kristin also wrote a Gratitude journal every day and focused on ten things she noticed she could do that day and consciously celebrated them. She was using all the FEARLESS resources and appropriate nonverbal signals, consistently, and got healthy.

It is normal to have remnants of old habits that had been established during illness. Just be like Kristin, STOP - THINK - GO. Don't avoid triggers. Change your response to triggers. That's how people recover. Reward yourself, not with being safe but celebrate your freedom from limitations. Give yourself something that says well done! Remember, your reward centre needs a hit to mark the moment. Here is an example of what happened to me, and how I turned it around:

As I opened my front door to go out, my whole body went into a full-blown panic attack, my legs packed in and I fell to the floor, immobilised, but in a very heightened state of arousal. As I lay on my hall floor, I wondered what on earth had just happened to me. Knowing how the brain works, I was able to deduce that my protective brain had associated going outside with danger, so had called on the chimp and reptile. To be fair, there was a lot of evidence that going outside is dangerous; since becoming ill, I had regularly ended up in ambulances from collapsing outside because I was determined to keep going, even if I did boom and bust. The meerkat was busy registering all the bad experiences. So, I lay on the floor and decided to stop the inappropriate reaction. I talked out loud, to the amygdala with a calm, determined voice:

> "It is safe to go outside. I don't need you- I can do this. I have spent my life going outside; it is what I do. I have played outside every day as a child, gone to school, clubs, dance classes, walked the hills, gone to work a zillion times, gone to shops, theatres, travelled on buses, trains, boats and planes- it is what I do. Going outside is safe, it is fun, it is normal. I have had five bad experiences, and you are obsessing on them, when I have had millions of good experiences outside. You need to reset that going outside is safe. From now on, I'll take it a bit easier and gradually build up to health, but you are not going to get me stuck, prevent me from opening a door, or stop me in my tracks. I needed you to stop me in my

tracks in the beginning, to save me from destroying my body, but I don't need you now. I've got this. Thank you."

As I shifted focus, the amygdala got the message, and the body gradually settled, enabling me to slowly mobilise again. I took a step outside, triumphant and said, "see chimp and reptile, I don't need you". Then I took more steps and broke free. The protective brain will *always* turn off when it knows you are safe. I know that when I went to walk outside, I was not consciously thinking of danger, but the protective brain is always busy working in the background. This is the Battle of the Brains, and we must inhibit the instinctive responses with the higher brain. Just remember:

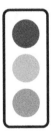

Stop.

Think, engage higher brain.

Proceed.

I know, if I had not taught health care and understood how the brain learns, I would have been terrified, become agoraphobic and housebound, like so many others. I would have shut the door and never wanted to go out again, because every time I tried, I would have had the same reaction. Just thinking about going outside would have given me the same response, because the brain can't differentiate between an abstract thought, and a real event.

In that moment, I felt for all the people with CFS who must have become terrified of symptoms, triggered by going outside, not knowing what to do to stop it. CFS groups and experts reinforce this by saying you will "pay for it if you do too much". They are kind and concerned, but they do not understand how the illness is being affected by conditioning to triggers. Instead, they just accept that "this is what happens with CFS "and tell you to adapt, by avoiding anything that makes you feel bad. The same is happening with Long Covid sufferers. You can fully recover when you break the survival response and thrive again.

Here is another true story to inspire you and to show how quickly you can turn things around:

> *Ben is a young 33-year-old man, who contracted Covid-19, and within a few weeks of the virus, he was housebound. It doesn't take long for the protective brain to take over.*
>
> *He had stopped all face-to-face contact with people, including his family as it was "too much". He explained that once he felt 80% better, he went for an hour walk but crashed for five days afterwards. He then learnt to reduce his activity to 30 minutes but still crashed, so by the time we spoke, he could only do 2 minutes, and the rest of the time, he was housebound, at home alone. Now, it seems logical to reduce activity if the activity caused the crash, and this is what the CFS Association, adaptive pacing therapy and specialists assume.*
>
> *However, it was the bad experience, caused by having a lowered threshold, that made the amygdala register that activity outside is dangerous. Like me at my front door, it made him avoid going out. Thankfully, Ben now knows not to give in to this – he recorded how many steps he can do indoors, and so rationally, how many he would therefore be able to do outdoors, when the chimp isn't in charge. Initially, he started by walking around his garden, to feel safe, and within a few days was "walking further than I have in a month". When you refuse to give in to the malfunctioning protective brain, you will thrive.*

Isn't it extraordinary that experts aren't curious that housebound patients can walk hundreds of steps indoors but not outdoors? When you notice that your body is reacting, whether because it has reached the reduced tolerance level or whether it is has become a conditioned response, please stay calm, and remind your protective brain that you are safe and take control. You can use these examples to help you. When the body is feeling okay, use it with confidence, rise above it and let your higher self, run the show.

Doing the Traffic Lights Procedure

THE RED is STOP. It is a pause to give the slow, clever brain time to kick in. Say STOP calmly, determined and in control, using a nonverbal gesture you would naturally use if you were meaning stop/enough. Refer to your nonverbal figures provided earlier.

AMBER is THINK. Engage the rational higher brain. Practise saying statements that resonates with you, such as:

- I don't need the animal brain. It doesn't serve me, and it is not useful.
- I am not going to let the protective brain control my life.
- I can override the chimp and the reptile and know I am safe.
- I will get my body working again.
- I will decide how I want to react.
- I can do this. I will pick myself back up, I did it before, and I'll do it again.
- I will do everything confidently, sensibly, joyfully, rationally, and mindfully.

Practise saying something that means you are back in control.

The human body is always trying to conserve energy. Habits and instincts are brilliantly efficient ways for the brain to function because they happen a hundred times faster than conscious decisions and are effortless, requiring little energy. Therefore, we run in autopilot most of the time, even when it isn't useful. The higher, conscious brain needs an awful lot of energy and effort to function, which is why we should take breaks when working and when putting in the effort to recover.

GREEN is PROCEED. Now you understand what is happening, you will change your conditioned response to everything just as Kristin, Ben and I did, and break free! You don't need the over-protective chimp and reptile anymore. Look back regularly at Kristin and Ben's stories to remind yourself of the right way to do it. Whatever triggered you, use the Traffic Lights system to stop reactions, take control and respond in a healthy way instead. Like Ben and Kristin, you can choose to reset to thrive, when faced with any reasonable activity. It will become a way of life again as you practise healthy connections. Be at ease in everything you do, not just your ten minutes breathing session. That's what we mean by being consistent. Be in the right state for doing activity and if you believe you can only manage one or two steps when climbing your stairs, that's great. Do something achievable then build on it. You are focused on associating previous triggers, such as hills or going outside, with successful outcomes. Once you are familiar with the Traffic Lights procedure, we will add another element to it in the next chapter, to speed your recovery.

The other E in BETTER is for Enjoying activity and movement

You can do an activity with fear and trepidation, in which case you will sabotage the outcome, or you can do an identical activity with joy, confidence, and fearlessness and get a much better outcome. Don't ever push through because that wouldn't be sensible but do be excited when you do anything, whether it is noticing you can make your own lunch, make a cup of tea, or go for a walk. You will put the evidence in your Recovery Journal.

It is essential to do exercises that you enjoy. A recent study showed that people who did activities they enjoyed "significantly improved their cortisol levels and ability to wake refreshed. People who didn't enjoy the event became worse because they found the event stressful or it felt like a chore, an effort, rather than pleasure." (Mosley et al, 2018). An activity must be nurturing to activate the vagal system and heal the body. These findings support the work by Selye, Sapolsky, McEwan, Naviaux, David Hamilton, Bruce Lipton, Candice Pert and many others, all of whom demonstrate how our world physically affects us. Have you noticed that when you are enjoying something, the body starts to settle? Find an activity you love, like gardening, which makes you focus on the plants rather than on yourself. Come up with options that require movement and that bring you joy.

A Meditation Exercise to Enjoy the Energy Flowing Within

This is a lovely exercise to energise and once you feel energised, decide what you would like to do that is enjoyable. I did this meditation every day, outside whenever possible, and then I would go for my manageable walk or dance to music. It is a great meditation to get grounded; so many people with CFS live in their heads with thoughts, both creative and destructive, constantly whirling. It is also a meditation to do if you are bedridden or wheelchair bound, putting strength back into your core and your legs. This meditation is adapted from the book, *M.E. (Chronic Fatigue Syndrome) and the Healer Within* (1993) by Nick Bamforth, which helped me a lot, during my recovery from CFS. It is useful to record the breathing and meditation exercises on your phone, so you can listen to them rather than read them.

1. Sit quietly outside if possible, or by a window, and close your eyes. Using your preferred breathing exercise, focus on your spinal cord, feeling the breath moving through it, then gradually extend your cord towards the earth. Imagine your cord as the roots of a tree going deep into the earth or it could be a rope or an anchor, grounding you to the earth, whatever you want it to be. Feel it travelling to the earth's core, going deeper, and getting warmer as you access the incredible energy from nature. Feel what it feels like to be so grounded, so steady, and still. Now notice channels of energy rising through your feet, rising through your legs and into your torso, filling you with a magnificent strength, and if you want to, give the energy a colour, a shape, or a sound. Notice the flow forming a circle, going up through your feet, and the overflow pours back into

the earth through your spine, giving eternal energy. And now, as this continuous energy flows, lift your attention to your head and notice as you lift your head to the sky, a gentle lightness from the universe pours through the top of your crown, washing away anything that isn't healthy as it flows into your body, your arms, light and soft. Let this beautiful golden light enter your heart, your lungs, healing any pain and flowing on into your vital organs, into your gut and your immune system. And sit for a moment, feeling what it feels like to have these different energies from nature: the grounded, solid energy from the earth and the light energy from the universe. As you feel the energy within, take a moment to enjoy it, and then, when you are ready, open your eyes and embrace the day. Lift your head to the sky and give gratitude for this moment and be curious what you might like to do now, that is enjoyable and revitalises you, letting you thrive.

This is a similar exercise for you to enjoy, to get grounded and to re-energise you, in preparation for using your body:

1. Sit comfortably, stand, or lie down, whichever is most comfortable for you. Settle into your breathing and step into what it feels like to be a living tree, any tree of your choosing; an oak tree in the middle of a field is often a favourite. Imagine being that tree. Feel the strength and stability of the tree, its stillness as it breathes in and out. Breathe in the joy of nature and breathe out gratitude, lifting your canopy to the sky. Notice your body rooted to the ground - feel what it feels like to be as grounded as a tree, connected, attached. Feel the energy coming up through your roots into your core being, filling you with this solid, earthy strength, keeping you grounded and your trunk sturdy. Look up to the sky and feel the air filtering through your upper limbs, raising your canopy to the sun, drawing in its warmth and vitality. Lift your head in gratitude for this day. Feel the lightness of the air as you breathe and let that breath spread through every cell in your being, filling you with vitality and energy. If you like, give it a symbol, a sound, or a colour, as you feel every cell in your body awakening. Enjoy this moment, and

just whenever you are ready, open your eyes and smile, thankful for another day and decide what you want to do today that is enjoyable.

R in BETTER is for Rest and Restore

Finally, life is about balance and harmony, so it is healthy to rest. Do not rest for the sake of it when you are feeling fine and energised, as recommended by the Action for M.E. pacing programme. Rest when your body wants a break. Learn to listen to your body and recognise when it is good to rest.

Restorative rest is when you feel at ease and at peace, relaxed and carefree. To do it otherwise, isn't rest; it is just lying down horizontally, in a bad state, activating the malfunctioning protective system.

It is essential to get into the habit of having breaks; stop for a break mid-morning, lunchtime, mid-afternoon and after dinner. Healthy people know how to balance work, rest, and play as part of their lifestyle. Do you know how to relax and be completely at ease, relaxing?

As mammals, we are born to rest as much as we are to move; lions have no problem with resting, so practise getting back into the natural rhythm of things. When we were younger, there were many times you enjoyed just chilling. If you notice you have an issue with resting because you have gremlins sitting on your shoulder saying, "rest is lazy", "other people will think I am lazy", or thinking that "rest means fatigue is back" then just notice them with serenity, stop and laugh at yourself for having these little gremlins, then do your Traffic Lights; stop, tell them they are not useful, and proceed-refocus on having healthy restorative rest.

Restorative Sleep. Your body's natural healer. If you notice that sleep is a problem for you, get into healthy sleep patterns. The more you practise healthy routines, the quicker you will return to normal. There is a high correlation between sleep deprivation or non-restorative sleep, and CFS. Furthermore, it is important to regulate your circadian cycle because irregular sleep patterns imbalance the hypothalamus and all the vital organs it controls.

- Have a regular sleep time routine, so the body realises it is downtime. Get rid of all light, mobiles, and laptops, including backlit kindles at least 40 minutes before going to bed, because the light inhibits melatonin, which is essential for sleep.
- Ensure the room is airy and at the right temperature for you.
- Do not have any caffeine after 6pm, if you have it at all. Research has shown that some people are much more susceptible to caffeine than others; if you take caffeine at noon, a quarter is still in your body at midnight.
- Read, listen to a story, or have an app like Headspace, to wind down. There are many apps available to help you sleep, which offer meditative music, white noise and sounds to relax you.
- If you are nocturnal or late sleeping, bring bedtime forward by 15 minutes and over time, keep adjusting it by another 15 minutes. Your circadian cycle is disrupted when survival mode is on, so you may notice you are now programmed to sleep midday and mid-morning. This will correct itself as you do the work to reset the system.
- Whatever is concerning you, tell yourself, "I can do nothing about it at this time of night, so I will package it up, and put it all into tomorrow. For now, I am going to count my blessings, focus on my successes and focus on my comfy bed, feeling the mattress, the pillow, and the duvet." Notice how you are shielded from the wind and the weather outside, cosy, and warm in bed. It is true that when you go to sleep counting your blessings, you have a better chance of sleep because stress chemicals keep you in arousal. Have a Gratitude Journal by your bed and write ten things in it before lying down or recite ten things.
- Consciously practise slowing your mind down by imagining waves getting smaller and fading. If you notice it racing again, that's okay, just visualise changing big waves into gentle sleep waves. Imagine a millpond that has been disturbed by a stone thrown into the middle of it, then just watch, mesmerised, as the ripples gently fade away.
- Never lie in bed frustrated or worried about not getting enough sleep as that just arouses the chimp and keeps you awake!
- If you cannot sleep, the current sleep recommendation is to get out of bed, to break the association that "bed means tossing and

turning". It's amazing and humbling to recognise how similar humans are to Pavlov's dogs, unconsciously hardwiring things together that happen at the same time. Break the state, move to another room, have a drink, read, and settle until you are tired enough to return to bed. Bed is only for sleep or enjoyable resting.

- You can rest in bed, even though you are not asleep. This is perfectly good, as restorative rest is better than tossing and turning, and essential when you are bedridden.
- Getting your body moving during the day will adjust the circadian cycle naturally.
- If you wake up startled, wired and feeling ill, the quickest way to reactivate the vagal system is to take a short, warm shower, graduating the temperature to cold for about 20-30 seconds or as long as you feel you can. It is *essential* that you do your breathing exercises to prepare the body before entering the shower and whilst in the shower. Going into cold air or moving on the spot also helps restart the body.
- Many of my clients recommend Lloyds Sleeping Aid tablets, available over the counter.

Summary

You will need to read this chapter to know what the exercises are, but a summary to trigger your memory and to look at regularly, is as follows. To correct this neurological malfunction and reactivate the healthy vagal system, remember to use FEARLESS:

Focus. Notice when your body can and does work for you. Record this in your journal or audio.

Excited. Emphasise successes and positive emotions.

Adapt. Your body will function according to the environment it is in. Practise finding achievable successes within your environment. Break unhealthy connections to triggers and reconnect activity to your healthy system.

Resilience. Keep bouncing back and be determined to get back on track, especially after a setback. Be rational and calm.

Love and Care for yourself. Get nurturing support from others.

Emotionally Detach from symptoms and do calm mindfulness.

Serenity, courage, gratitude, and amazing grace.

See Things Differently. Change your perception of triggers- they are just neutral things. Symptoms are just sensations. Your body can heal when the amygdala detects everything is safe.
CONSISTENCY is the key to recovery. Become FEARLESS as a way of life, not just as an exercise.

Remember that the ventral vagus nerve attaches to your lungs and heart, so breathe from the diaphragm. Do the exercises with a smile, and an uplifted tone of voice. It is not what you do, it's the way that you do it.

Use your body to reactivate the healthy, healing vagal system. Use the acronym BETTER just like you do with FEARLESS and have these acronyms handy and visible to keep you on track.

BETTER is:

Breathing exercises and meditation.

Exercise the body. Use your body, through doing reasonable activity, to activate the vagal system.

Throat exercises. Gargle, blow, sing, chant, hum, to activate the vagus nerve.

Traffic Lights. Stop being triggered into automatic responses, take control, engage your rational brain, and choose how you want to proceed to get into a healthy state.

Enjoy. Only do exercises that you enjoy and that turn on thrive mode.

Rest peacefully between periods of mobilising. Relax, take breaks, and improve your restorative sleep.

Chapter 6:
Easing the Bumpy Road
To Recovery

Three people start on a journey of a thousand miles. The first one begins by saying "I will never be able to do this". The second says "what if we can, just one step at a time" and the third man starts, but gives up at the first hurdle. Which one is likely to complete the journey? – A saying that was coined by Jan, and one she found extremely useful in terms of her recovery.

Saboteurs and Gremlins

- Check out if anything is holding you back from recovery. The saboteurs in this chapter are all related by clients who had been struggling.

- Are you prioritising recovery or trying to keep going for others? Why? This illness is serious. Your whole body is being shut down, and you cannot function, so please take it seriously. Many people end up bedridden for life, in care homes and some even die, so do what you would do if it were another serious illness.

- If you don't take it seriously, others won't appreciate how bad you are. If you seem okay, then of course others will let you carry on.
- Do you feel useless and judged if you need to lie down? Please, for now, suspend every useless belief /opinion and prioritise health. Other people want you to be healthy.
- If you are preoccupied with being the doer, the provider, I empathise, but it is not useful for recovery. I was devastated at the prospect of losing my job and our home, but my children said, "Mum, we don't care if we live in a caravan, as long as you are healthy". As adults, we lose sight of what matters because we become driven by adulting, being carers and providers; it takes a child to remind us that health is our number one priority. There are no prizes for being the brave soldier pushing through and it is detrimental during recovery to be thinking about responsibilities. Focus only on recovery.

Jake's Story

One lovely young man, Jake, had been stuck for a few years, boom and busting, where he often got back to work, then crashed again, back in bed. When he crashed, he became frustrated and desperate and then went back to work too soon because he was self-employed and every day, he worried about his business going under and paying the bills. He had no idea why his body wasn't working for him. When we spoke, we realised he had become a slave to his business and he had to be prepared to let go. Yes, this is a tall order, but the alternative is to keep doing the same old pattern and become more ill. Once he accepted that he might lose his business and his home, he focused only on recovery, telling his clients he had suspended business for now and would reconnect as soon as possible. By becoming detached from anything that didn't aid recovery, he was able to heal." When he fully committed to recovering, he did recover.

During recovery he realised that his business had been a weight on him for so long. He had found conflict with customers impossible and so he had accommodated their every demand, often finishing work for free or in the evenings. During recovery, his business had to go on hold, but he survived the worst and picked up the company again. Now, he knows, "If I can survive that, I can survive anything".

The experience taught him not to be concerned about getting business or losing customers, and he was humbled by how many customers cared about his health. During follow up sessions, he learnt how to deal with difficult customers and workload, just as you will learn in Part Two.

Jake had always wanted to recover but fear about losing his business meant he had kept pushing through when he wasn't back to full health, and that meant he kept crashing.

A major piece of research was carried out in 2002 on anxiety. It concluded that 70% of what we worry about never happens, and of the 30% that does happen, only 4% we find hard to deal with. With this in mind:

- Instead of catastrophising on what "might happen", focus on what is happening right now. Mindfulness is to fill your mind with what is useful and what is relevant, right now. Getting physically better is your job right now.
- Remember, all recipes for success follow the same process and need the same resources, FEARLESS and BETTER.
- Get rid of any expectation of when you will recover. How long is a piece of string? It doesn't matter, but there is an end to it. Just know you will recover.
- When your tolerance level is low, pressure will put you over the threshold and make you ill. Jake and others struggled as they were desperate to get back to work in two weeks or two months. Pressure increases demands, and you don't need more demands when your supply is low. Notice if you are feeling any pressure to recover, from others or from your own concerns and values. It is not useful as it will sabotage recovery. Your body is telling

you to look after yourself. You need to build your reserves first, and only then meet the demands. Take the pressure off and focus on recovery, one step at a time. Go to Citizen's Advice, food banks or any relevant sources to get support.

- Are you expecting symptoms to have gone, and get upset or give up if they return days, weeks or months later? Revise your expectations because recovery is not linear and people who recover know there will be ups and downs. The malfunctioning pattern has run in default for a long time, so it would be reasonable that it will take a while to reset it. The body needs time to recuperate when it has done more than usual; when people recover from heart attacks, pneumonia, strokes, or cancer, there are times when the body is exhausted and times when they feel as if symptoms are coming back.

Here is a graph for recovery. What do you see? Notice that there are always ups and downs in any recovery, and that you gradually go on an upward gradient, even though, on any particular day you can feel as if you have gone backwards.

For recovery, we notice that a downward period is always followed by an upturn; there is always another up. Hurrah! We focus on the ups and make the brain register the ups, whilst expecting there to be downs. We learn serenity and grace as we wait for the blip to pass and for the ups to come again. If you read the graph like this, then you are doing brilliantly. If you notice the downs and catastrophise about the downs, then you will get stuck and sabotage success, so you need to stop, and refocus on recovery and health. Refresh yourself on how you need to be approaching recovery:

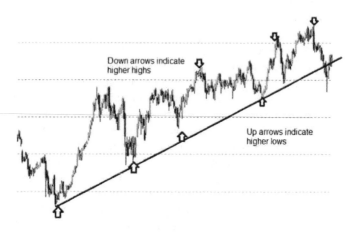

Down arrows indicate higher highs

Up arrows indicate higher lows

EXERCISE. Jot down all the resources we need to make healthy connections with activities and movement. Fill in what each letter means below:

F

E

A

R

L

E

S

S

Notice how much you are doing FEARLESS already, consistently throughout each day, and be really proud of yourself.

Now do the same for how to work your body, getting the healthy pathways reactivated. Do you remember the exercises and activities

suggested in the last chapter to make you BETTER?
Jot down what BETTER stands for.

B

E

T

T

E

R

- Expectation is so important in recovery. When we expect there to be downs, we are okay with it, we deal with it, and we stay on track. I know from experience how much expectation affects recovery. The first time I recovered, I dealt with crashes calmly and expected them to happen. The second time I took ill when I was referred to specialists, I saw crashes as proof that the experts must be right and was then tortured by thinking, "what if I don't recover?"
- If you boom and bust like Jake, meaning you do lots then crash, you may have unrealistic expectations. You assume you have recovered as soon as you feel good but will be shocked and devastated when symptoms return. In recovery, you need to expect symptoms will return for quite a while and, being fit to walk is not the same as being fit to work. The new twist on Traffic Lights at the end of this chapter will help speed up recovery and a return to normality.
- Do you feel shame or frustration about appearing weak during illness? Remember molecules of emotion physically change your body and being helpless, ashamed or depressed will maintain the malfunctioning system. Fear and shame can make you push through, even though you are ill. Are you ashamed to be thought of as weak? You are not weak; your body needed to stop because it was given a hammering that others didn't have. In my

experience, people with CFS and Long Covid are so mentally strong and determined to keep going that they didn't listen to their bodies.

- Pushing through and exposing yourself to activities that make you feel dreadful only serves to reinforce the Pavlovian responses you want to stop. Not useful or healthy.
- Are you still limiting your life to avoid triggers because it is "easier" to give in? Please do not get stuck. The extended Traffic Lights exercise will enable you to break patterns quickly.
- Watch your language, your tone of voice and how you are perceiving things, because they will tell you if you are in thrive or survive mode.

Sabotaging the Ups:

Here are examples of what people say when they are feeling better, which completely sabotages recovery:

- I knew it wouldn't last.
- I've had ups before, but I always crash.
- I'm feeling good but so scared that I'm going to do too much and crash.
- I feel better, but I'm always waiting for the payback.
- I could do the activity, but that doesn't mean I am better.
- I don't have any ups. I only notice downs.

Sabotaging Recovery When There Are Setbacks:

Likewise, here are some common statements from sufferers who will struggle to recover:

- It is too hard to keep picking yourself up again.
- I'm never going to get better.
- I am completely devastated. I thought I was getting better.
- I just have to accept that I can't recover.

- I did too much and now I've destroyed my body.
- I should have listened to the experts, who told me it is my fault for doing too much.
- I should have recovered by now. I can't do it.
- I am trapped in this body and terrified I have permanent damage.
- I knew I would pay for it. I'm having a payback day.

Notice how these unhealthy beliefs and responses cannot aid recovery. If you catch yourself thinking any of these things, it is entirely understandable, but it is not useful. Give yourself permission to be sad, to be devastated and upset, but then after 20 minutes, pick yourself up, and commit to being resilient and use your FEARLESS resourcefulness. Using the last few chapters, review what you need to do for ups and downs as you progress on the bumpy road to recovery, and using your FEARLESS resources and BETTER exercises.

- Do you have gremlins calling you lazy if you aren't busy, so you push through? Someone taught you that laziness is a sin. It isn't. A balanced life, including relaxation, is essential and sensible. Break free from the gremlins to thrive. You will use the Traffic Lights to overcome unhealthy patterns.
- How do you react if you are called selfish? Do you think looking after yourself and prioritising health is selfish? Somewhere you learnt that considering yourself is wrong. Whoever embedded that in you is wrong, and they are most likely wanting you to only focus on providing for their needs. Considering yourself is essential and healthy.
- If a part of you is resisting change, or habits are entrenched, then the online videos at www.resettothrive.co.uk will be useful, particularly the Partswork and Reimprinting techniques.

I also highly recommend Eye Movement Desensitisation and Reprocessing (EMDR) as a highly effective therapy for resolving past experiences that gets you stuck. It is clinically-trailed and used widely for specific or chronic trauma that impacts the body. Becoming debilitated with Long Covid or CFS is traumatic. You can also seek out a qualified coach; I would recommend Mark Lister, who offers a free 30-minute consultation, to increase your awareness of saboteurs and gremlins (www.markthecoach.wordpress.com). Also, Alan Mead is a wonderful person and coach, whose resources can be visited at www.alanmead.co.

You may find it useful to access a neurolinguistic programming (NLP) trainer who can take you through goal setting and accessing healthy states. Try www.lifecoach-directory.org.uk or www.nlpcoachfinder.com. Cat Paterson (www.catpaterson.co.uk), who features in the online *Reset to Thrive* programme, is a trained breathing expert. As a practitioner of Rapid Transformational Therapy (RTT), which combines the principles of hypnotherapy, NLP, psychotherapy, cognitive behavioural therapy, and neuroscience, she can help you break free of unconscious and unwanted saboteurs. Ensure any coach resonates with you, so you feel you can trust them.

A Quick Technique: Using Traffic Lights with Neuro Linguistic Programming (NLP)

Immediately after a virus such as Covid-19 or the onset of CFS, a long period of rest is essential. You cannot do a quick fix when your body needs time out. You have been pulverised, so stop, and accept your body needs to recuperate and look after yourself. During the first 3-6 months of being ill, master the FEARLESS tools and do BETTER exercises within your remit.

I recommend you only use this quick technique anytime you still notice symptoms after 3-6 months of becoming ill. This technique is used when your body is stuck and malfunctioning. Symptoms may still appear "out of the blue" when you thought you had recovered; but that's normal. You can use this technique to stop them and get back on track.

NB. I have purposefully not put this technique into the previous recovery chapters because you need to become proficient in all the FEARLESS resources to be able to do this "quick fix" successfully. You will not get the results you want unless you do it with a FEARLESS approach.

I recovered completely the first time I had ME/CFS, but I hadn't made the changes needed for permanent health, so had a relapse. The relapse enabled me to learn lessons about how to do life the right way and introduced me to this technique from Neuro Linguistic Programming

(NLP) called Associating into Healthy States; it quickly enables you to turn off the malfunctioning, protective system and activate the healthy vagal system, which helps restart the body.

FEARLESS and BETTER exercises return the body to the healthy state, and they are how I recovered the first time. The beauty of this additional technique is that you can use it when you are out and about and your body goes into over arousal or shutdown modes. If you find it difficult to take control of the protective brain over sustained periods, then this quick technique can be powerful for you. You can be confident to go out and about, knowing you have this tool to use any time you need it and then you carry on normally. Like the children's pop-up toy below, whenever symptoms pop back up again, you use this tool to knock them back down. Treat it as a handy tool you carry in your back pocket and can use whenever or wherever you need to.

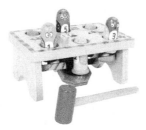

Associating into healthy states activates the vagal system, so the body switches on again – then you take it for granted it is working, so carry on as normal. The mantra is "If the body is working, it is normal, so do normal activities."

The Associating into Healthy states technique requires precision; it is easy to do it slightly wrong and get no results. I recovered the first time without it and when you master the ways described in this book, you can recover without it too. However, it definitely speeds up recovery when done right and is a great technique for breaking unhealthy patterns, as detailed in Part Two. Always remember the "Traffic Lights" procedure:

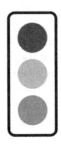

STOP, PAUSE

THINK: ENGAGE HIGHER BRAIN. TAKE CONTROL. DECIDE HOW YOU WANT TO BE

PROCEED IN A HEALTHY STATE.

Traffic Lights (TL) is a simple, well recognised procedure in health and social care practice. You are learning to stop automatic responses to triggers by doing a conscious override that uses the higher brain functions. You choose a healthy response and proceed safely. In behaviour centres, we trained young people to access social skills and anger management strategies on the green section of the traffic lights procedure (TL), so they could then proceed with their day in a better state.

Rather than proceed with BETTER exercises on the green section of TL, we will now use the NLP technique of associating into a healthy state to get the body working quickly. You would still use your FEARLESS and BETTER tools consistently in day-to-day life but use this as soon as symptoms appear. Instantly stop them and revert to normal. It's useful to have Traffic Lights displayed to remind you to use it. Have red, amber, green elastic bands on your wrist or dots on your hand. Put traffic lights everywhere!

Follow The Traffic Lights Procedure, incorporating the NLP technique

Awareness. By now you should be very aware of your triggers and your response to triggers. It may be your body reacting badly to opening a front door or shutting down after low level activity. When you notice unhealthy responses, use Traffic Lights and all your FEARLESS resources.

RED = STOP. Use your voice and nonverbal signals (NVS) to express a definite, firm, and compassionate stop. Never be scared or frustrated. Use a word that resonates with you; a client, who was a professional jockey used "wow" and as soon as he said it, the higher brain took control because it had learnt "wow" means control.

Look back at the diagrams on nonverbal signals and notice the facial expression and the gesture you would use. If you are using it because the body is shutting down, your nonverbal signals need to look and sound energised. If you are feeling wired or over aroused, use a very slow, calm approach. Your breathing will be from the diaphragm, so slow and gentle.

AMBER = THINK & ENGAGE YOUR CONSCIOUS BRAIN. Talk to yourself in a kind way, thinking about what you are saying. Say the same thing each time, so it becomes automatic, quicker, like any habit. This is what I say, but choose something that resonates with you about taking control:

> "This is not useful.
> Focus, Breathe.
> Come on, you *can* do this.
> How do you need to be right now?
> Healthy, strong, back to normal."

Say it like you mean it. Be confident that you can get yourself better; you have been making changes already, so any doubt is simply just the chimp chattering away. Ignore it. The focus gesture is useful for getting you focused on the exercise. On amber, you are consciously making judgements, decisions, and choices, and building your confidence. Be calmly rational; no panicking or shouting chimps. Record yourself on your mobile phone to check that you look and sound in control. You have been practising the FEARLESS resources, so you can do this successfully.

GREEN = USING THE NLP TECHNIQUE TO ASSOCIATE INTO A HEALTHY STATE. For now, we are going to use this technique to access a healthy body. Later, you will use it to access the appropriate state you need at any given moment.

Compose yourself, take a breath and use your focus gesture, whether it's the blinkered horse or the single hand going straight as an arrow from the nose forward. Say "focus" to commit one hundred percent to the exercise; *nothing else matters* for the few moments you are doing the exercise. Take yourself to a quiet place- the loo is great, as you can lock the door.

When you master this technique, you can learn to do it in company and anytime you need it; the online *Reset to Thrive* course demonstrates a subtle version often used by elite sports people and presenters prior to performing. If you are not getting results, stop and review. You do not want to practise bad habits. This exercise activates the healthy vagus nerve by firing off healthy associations, our Pavlovian responses. Attached to every memory are thousands of neural connections that act like a constellation of stars, firing off sensations and feelings. We want to fire off the healthy connections and reactivate the healthy body.

- Close your eyes and take yourself back to anytime when your body did work for you, a good moment. You probably had a few moments of well-being recently or choose a great moment from anytime in your life. Make the brain remember, so it can fire off the healthy pathways again.
- To access energy, find a moment when your body is moving and feels amazing. Everything about this moment is healthy; how you are feeling, thinking, being, responding. (If you need to bring the body down from arousal or pain, then find a really calm, powerful moment, and again do all the NVS relevant in this moment.)
- FOCUS. Really step into that moment, noticing everything. Get into the posture, use the exact tone of voice, facial expression,

gestures, and notice the position of your head. If you are walking, actually feel your body walking and get into its rhythm and pace, making tiny movements on the spot. Have the gestures and actions exactly as you are right now in this healthy moment.

- In the present, notice what you are seeing, hearing, touching, smelling and tasting. Fire off the sensory input associated with this healthy moment. Make your brain register you are there, right now. Be aware of what it feels like in this moment, notice where you feel it and how your body feels in this healthy moment. Let it spread to every part of you.

- As soon as you access the healthy state, add a colour, a shape, a sound, a song, or click your fingers. Find something to associate with this peak moment. Symbols are like the bell to the food, in Pavlovian response. When you associate them enough times, you can automatically access health, just by bringing up symbols.

- Take your mind off this moment; think about cabbages! Bring up your symbol and notice how quickly you feel the healthy state.

As you open your eyes, notice that you have won the Battle of the Brains. You have overcome the chimp and the reptile and fired off the healthy human pathways again. Let the chimp have a rest, as you become more resourceful. Feel how wonderful it is to Break Free!

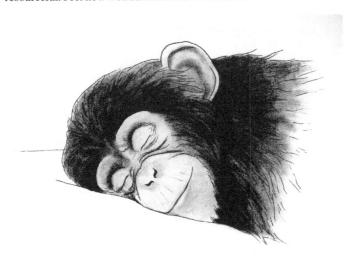

You are now a very resourceful person, equipped with the knowledge, understanding and tools to achieve your goal and recover! Amble along and feel proud of yourself!

If you notice that you have been out of practise with FEARLESS resources, this Traffic Light procedure can really help you access the resources again. For instance, during this exercise, you may notice that you are focused on symptoms, so you need to practise your emotional detachment from anything that isn't useful and see symptoms as just odd sensations that will stop when you focus fully on the healthy moment. Be mindful of any saboteurs and be fascinated that these gremlins have crept up on you, unnoticed, then watch the *Reset to Thrive* videos to master the technique. Use Traffic Lights to step into a moment when you are:

- Focused.
- Excited.
- Adapt the body naturally by letting it know you are OKAY, and that your world is safe.
- Resilient and rational. You can do this.
- Love yourself enough to look after yourself.
- Emotionally detached from symptoms and neutral events.
- Serene and courageous.
- Seeing things differently. The world is safe, and I am okay. Stairs are just stairs. Outside is freedom. Symptoms are just sensations.

You may need to find separate moments for each resource, but one moment can access several resources. For instance, a moment when you gave a presentation or chatted about an event could invoke focus, enthusiasm, resilience, and emotional detachment. You will become familiar with this technique in Part 2, as you use it to access however you need to be in any given moment.

Summary

The road to recovery will have ups and downs and that is normal; expect it. Go back to the list of gremlins and saboteurs to check there is nothing getting in the way of moving forward. Ben, Kirstin and I changed our response to triggers by using the Traffic Lights procedure to engage the rational higher brain and override our primal instincts and habits.

You can also use an extended version of the Traffic Lights, incorporating an NLP technique, to access the resources in the FEARLESS toolkit and for getting your body back to normal. It takes practise to learn a new skill, so take time to master this traffic lights version. Keep reviewing the Traffic Light (TL) section and watch demonstrations online at www.resettothrive.co.uk.

Part Two: Post Recovery – Staying Healthy

Chapter 7: Making Your Environment Healthy

Every living organism thrives in a nurturing habitat,
but barely survives in harsh conditions.

The Relapse

I was so ecstatic when I recovered - I had such a zest for life and was fit and healthy for four years from that point on. However, I had gone straight back to spinning even more plates and was still physically affected by people behaving badly. I was bullied at work from my line manager but couldn't get support from higher up. In private life, one woman, who swore she would destroy me and my husband, provided relentless, ongoing chronic stress and burden, so there was little reprieve to buffer against this 24/7 overload. Compounding this was my emotional overload, and watching my lovely mum die a horrible death from cancer. This triggered endless nightmares and terrible sleep deprivation that carried on for a long time. On top of this, lacking sleep, grieving, managing a behaviour centre and having a To Do List that lasted from 6.30 am till after midnight almost every day meant I eventually succumbed again to viruses. But being the conscientious worker, I kept pushing through, with flu-like symptoms so that students wouldn't be disadvantaged in their up-and-coming exams. Ironically, I could deal with constant conflict and discord in my role and managing a behaviour centre but was physically shaken by conflict and powerlessness in my private life - that's the power of triggers and Pavlovian conditioning. The first sign of the relapse was having excruciating pain when the curtains were opened, letting in summer sun - my husband laughed, calling me Dracula, but whilst I laughed, I knew something was wrong. A few weeks later, in the middle of my To Do List, I was walking the dog, feeling absolutely fine and happy, then, 300 metres from home, I just ground to a halt. It all happened in less than a minute. It took nearly an hour to complete the walk and then I was back in bed. Again.

At the time, I was utterly devastated; I had removed myself from a situation that I knew had led to my illness, I lived with lovely people and never imagined I would be ill again. When I relapsed, I was referred to the CFS specialist team. The shock of getting ME/CFS back and then being told by the CFS Team that I would never recover left me distraught, thinking maybe the consultant was right when he told me I was "lucky to have periods of remission". The thought of living like this was depressing. Hopelessness and helplessness are not ingredients for recovery and do get us stuck. I listened to the specialists' prognosis, and started to doubt myself, but a part of me could never accept their insistence that we can't recover, because I had recovered before on my own, so must be able to recover again. The first time, I had consistently used all the healthy FEARLESS resources, did my BETTER vagal exercises, and used my body when it felt well. This time, I fluctuated between the conviction that I can and the fear that I can't, going one step forward and two steps back.

Having done it both ways, I know that it takes 100% conviction to recover, and stay focused on recovery, because doubt gets us stuck in a downward spiral. I also learnt how important it is to be consistent. During the relapse, professionals were telling me, "It's your fault you are crashing, you do too much. You must accept you can't recover; you were just lucky the first time". I was even told I needed to grieve for the person I had been because she has gone forever! Despair replaced serenity and sabotaged recovery. Whilst I tried to ignore their advice and made progress, their conviction bore into me, so a part of me was terrified they were right, and this sabotaged recovery. The first time,

I was utterly focused, and I knew I could recover and was consistent.

Thankfully, I found someone who reminded me that I can recover and guided me through my relapse. It is useful to have someone to encourage you and who understands that you can recover. The relapse also introduced me to the neurolinguistic programming technique of Associating into Healthy States, which was critical for changing embedded patterns that I had been running for a lifetime. I made a full recovery but lost my job because the occupational doctor followed NICE guidelines, saying there is no cure, and I would relapse in future. Sadly, I still didn't change anything about my lifestyle.

It was only when I knew I was going under for a third time a few years later that I made a life changing decision. The possibility of another relapse forced me to review my life. My mantra was "Nothing and nobody is ever going to bring me down again". I would never have CFS again.

It isn't enough to get physically better and go back doing the same old ways. I had to learn to set boundaries so I couldn't be overloaded, and I had to live in a nurturing environment. Even though setting boundaries and saying no to unreasonable demands led to discord, then loss and grief, it was worth it to stay healthy. Most importantly for me, and so many others, I needed to learn to be unaffected by other peoples' unhealthy patterns or anger, regardless of who they are.

I believe that for many people who have been ill, Part Two is essential for permanent recovery. No more relapses! The adaptive survival system will never turn on if the environment is nurturing, when demands are manageable, and supplies are robust. If you have ever had a relapse, become mindful of your environment, demands and your resourcefulness.

Staying Healthy After Recovery

Here are just a few things you may want to consider. To stay in the calm, thrive mode (our green track), we need to meet the demands of life. To do this we have to:

- Reduce the number of demands and load, and don't turn on rocket fuels to keep us going.
- Increase our supplies, our resourcefulness.

- Have a clear perception of realistic demands.
- Live in a healthy environment with supportive, nurturing people.
- Deal with viruses or infection in the future.
- Develop a healthy sleep pattern and restorative rest.

In this chapter, we look at decreasing the demands and load in your life, so you stay healthy in future. The next chapter looks at increasing your resourcefulness.

By reducing demands and increasing supply, we can naturally bridge the gap between supply and demand, and not rely on the chimp to mobilise us.

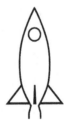

DEMANDS. Rocket fuels are only needed when the gap is too great.

SUPPLY. When Supply can meet demands easily, you will be healthy.

Firstly, let's review how we are meant to function in our natural world. By now, you will have noticed that a central theme in this book is that the body lives in a healthy physiology when it is in a good place, but it switches into survival physiology when it detects that life is hard and conditions are unfavourable. You know by now that this process occurs automatically via your adaptive system (ANS). When our environment and our lifestyle is not healthy, demands outweigh supply. With CFS and Long Covid, eventually the reptile shut us down and we got stuck in this protective mode. Demands were even harder as we pushed through with a body that had been reset to a very low threshold. Furthermore, being exposed to activities in this bad state meant neutral events got filed as threats and so we were constantly triggered back into protective mode.

It is so important to recognise how our physiology and well-being is affected by our environment. You are either thriving or surviving. Neutrality is part of thriving and is when you are cruising along and feeling at ease. Adaptation means we biologically adapt to our surroundings; if we live in a toxic environment, we will struggle. Like any living organism on the planet, we must live in a habitat that suits us and is suitable for us. Once you are fully recovered, notice if your habitat is healthy for sustained wellbeing. Are you in a place where you feel at ease and can thrive? Is there anything about demands that may be unreasonable or unmanageable? Now is a time to consider how you need your physical world to be. I learnt I need peace, nature, space, me time, a loving, stable home, good friends, and support. What nurtures you? For instance, if you are creative, are you ensuring that your lifestyle enables you to express this need?

It is not just the physical environment; we know that a lack of social support and unhealthy attachments are just as stressful to mammals and humans (Harlow 1958; Bowlby, and Ainsworth, 1992). As Julianne Holt-Lunstad writes in Health Affairs):

> Cumulative meta-analytical evidence indicates that poor social connection increased risk of developing heart disease by 29 percent and risk for stroke by 32 percent. Although fewer studies examine other outcomes, there is also evidence that poorer social connection is associated with poorer general health and well-being, as well as with newly and previously diagnosed type 2 diabetes. Social connection and isolation even influence the probability of developing a cold, independent of baseline immunity, demographics, and health practices. (21st June 2020)

Social and emotional attachment are the most significant buffers against stress. Therefore, your environment needs to have social and emotional support to stay healthy.

Pause for a moment and consider if you have sufficient support, emotionally, socially, and in terms of sharing the physical load. When we lose sight of how nature intended us to live, our lifestyle becomes unsustainable, and our body gets out of balance.

Adapting to occasional stressors is fine and healthy, even exciting and stimulating. Challenges give us a buzz and make us feel alive.

But over time, living in an environment that is not healthy will cause chronic overuse of the survival adaptive system, causing illnesses, or chronic fatigue syndrome. Anyone can deal with problems some of the time, but no one can live with them constantly. Furthermore, as resourceful people, we can deal with all sorts of problems, but there are times in people's lives when too many things come at us all at once; then demands outweigh supply. Had you been bombarded by too many things hitting the fan all at the same time? A virus on top of grief, loss, excessive workload, or relationship problems? Have a think about your own individual situation and whether these are now resolved.

How Overload Contributes to Chronic Fatigue Syndrome, Long Covid and Post Viral Fatigue Syndrome

In Chapter 2 we looked at how every structure on the planet has a tolerance level, beyond which it will start to show stresses, strains, or breakdown. All structures in nature, and in engineering, are built to withstand a certain load. Materials show fatigue if they are taken beyond their tolerance level, and the human body experiences breakdown when it likewise goes beyond its natural tolerance level. Research shows that the body starts to fluctuate and struggle under duress.

> *"This does not involve a malfunction per se. Even the most finely tuned stress response in the healthiest of individuals can begin to cause damage, if activated again and again over a long period. In other words, chronic stress can cause illness... Chronic stress can take a toll on the immune system, making someone more susceptible to colds and infections. It can also ratchet up the immune response to detrimental levels, resulting in allergies, asthma, and autoimmune conditions... and other stress-related illnesses including colitis, chronic fatigue syndrome, fibromyalgia, eczema. The stress response musters the brain, glands, hormones, immune system, heart, blood, and lung. Hence the array of illnesses that can arise when we get stressed".* (McEwan 2002 p.21).

Stress is not about being emotionally overwhelmed; stress is physical damage to the body when bombarded with unreasonable, excessive demands. Load can be the drip, drip, drip effect we experience over many years, or it can be being bombarded with too many unpredictable problems all at the same time.

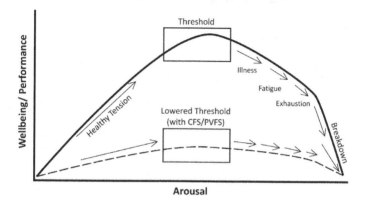

Had you experienced any relentless long term social discord, isolation, or physical and emotional overload before succumbing to a virus? During the illness, everything is overload because we are functioning at a low threshold with limited reserves.

As McEwan says in the above quote, "Even the most finely tuned stress response in the healthiest of individuals can begin to cause damage if activated again and again over a long period." This means that we were perfectly healthy people and responded normally to exceptional, long-term load. Only you truly know your circumstances and life experiences and only you can change them.

Overload has got nothing to do with mental health or a personality problem; it is simply having too much for any human to deal with. It is nobody's fault, and you are not to blame, but recognising unhealthy factors in our environment gives us the opportunity to make life better. Our bodies are the most complicated, brilliant, magical machinery ever created, but all mechanisms go wrong when overused.

We can break the load, or demands, into several sections and use a simple acronym to guide us: **PIES.**

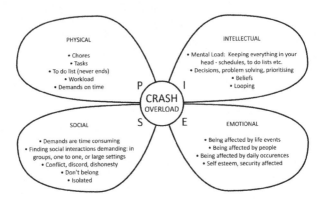

Becoming Loaded with P.I.E.S.

PHYSICAL
• Chores
• Tasks
• To do list (never ends)
• Workload
• Demands on time

INTELLECTUAL
• Mental Load: Keeping everything in your head - schedules, to do lists etc.
• Decisions, problem solving, prioritising
• Beliefs
• Looping

CRASH OVERLOAD

SOCIAL
• Demands are time consuming
• Finding social interactions demanding: in groups, one to one, or large settings
• Conflict, discord, dishonesty
• Don't belong
• Isolated

EMOTIONAL
• Being affected by life events
• Being affected by people
• Being affected by daily occurences
• Self esteem, security affected

Physical: viruses, infections, operations, activity, chores, workload, time pressures, our To Do Lists, sleep deprivation, irregular circadian cycle, keeping going too long, poor diet, excessive exercise.

Intellectual: keeping everything in your head; the to-do list, decisions, tasks, memorising dates and appointments, problems, problem solving, multi-tasking, learning new things, learning challenging information.

Emotional: Trauma, loss, and grief. Life events, such as transitioning to a new place, a school or secondary school. Being affected by situations, other people, and concerns about our self-image or having low self-esteem. Can include fear, frustration, anger, arousal, anxiety, guilt, blame, shame, feeling inferior, powerless, upset, hurt, shock, embarrassment, disgust.

Social demands: accommodating others, keeping others happy, rejection or fear of rejection, keeping the peace, fear of missing out, social anxiety, juggling events, expectations, criticism, judgements, comparing ourselves to others, conflict, discord, bullying, cultural norms, isolation.

Again, the key points here are sustainability and timing. When you look at this list, were the demands ongoing, never ending, or did too many things come at you all at once? Often clients use the word overwhelmed to express overload. Start to notice when you feel overwhelmed as this is a good indicator for overload. Enthusiasts may not notice they are overwhelmed because they feast on life, or they become so mentally focused on keeping going that they ignore signs from the body that they need to rebalance. Overwhelmed does not mean anxious; it is literally your body being overloaded.

We all know that overdoing it for years impacts on health. That's why when people have a heart attack, cancer, or another illness, we talk about "having had a warning sign and needing to take it easier." It shouldn't take for us to be seriously ill to learn a balanced life, but our society prides itself on keeping going and being industrious. We lose sight of what it takes to be healthy, then live on a wing and a prayer, hoping we will survive another day.

P in PIES stands for Physical Overload

Workload, Chores and To Do Lists. As we saw in the previous quote from McEwan, overload will make us susceptible to viruses, illnesses, and infection, and so it is essential to look at what was overloading you. Were you literally keeping going for hours because you "had to get things done"? Listen out for your language. If you hear yourself saying I "have to" or "got to", then there is a good chance you feel you have no control over your load.

You can do this for a while, even years, but it is not sustainable. Are you expected to constantly learn new skills, process new information, and get up to speed quickly in your role? That takes a lot of effort and energy.

In an article, "How Millennials Became the Burnout Generation", Anne Helen Petersen (2020) explains that "adulting" is a word invented by millennials as a catchall for the tasks of self-sufficient existence. She writes, "to adult, is to complete your to-do list - but everything goes on the list, and the list never ends." They are forever struggling to catch up and failing. Millennials have "errand paralysis", paralysed by the thought of having to deal with another thing to do. As Petersen says, "this burnout is not a temporary affliction: it's the millennial condition. It's our base temperature. It's the way things are. It's our lives".

Does this concept of adulting resonate with you? Did you feel overloaded with endless tasks, responsibilities and problems but always feeling like you were doing catch up? Millennials were brought up to optimise and to keep optimising. Both genders are often overloaded with endless tasks, although a recent report on lockdown data shows that, in households with a child aged under 5 years, women did on average 78% more childcare than men and women did more than double the proportion of cooking, childcare and housework than men. This gender gap narrowed to just 20% with children aged 5 to 10-years. (ONS 2020)

It is not only this generation who struggle though. The whole of history is littered with certain cohorts being so overloaded they couldn't function; illness and early death was the norm in historical times. A more modern example came with the Baby Boomer generation and the rise of feminism and the contraceptive pill. Women were told they should be able to do it all, that they should be the perfect mum, partner, career woman, sex-bomb and all-round sport. Women in particular ended up doing full-time jobs, full-time childcare and were full-time housekeepers. What was initially liberating became unreasonable, with many women becoming overloaded with three full-time jobs and mentally overloaded with an enormous To Do List. Furthermore, they were made to feel guilty if they were "only housewives" or if they complained about their 24/7 workloads, which only added to their emotional and social overload.

Liberation has been a double-edged sword for many, both empowering and exhausting. Like every transition, it created discord, as men felt challenged or disempowered, unwilling to share the household and parenting roles with their working partner. Many relationships felt the strain, so social, physical, mental, and emotional overload increased.

What is making people push so hard? Our values and morals are entrenched and unconscious; we rarely think about them, but we are utterly driven by them. They are at the core of who we are, our identity.

They don't have to be stated; children learn by watching, listening and role modelling. Millennials grew up with unrealistic expectations and values to always optimise. In his book *Man Down: Why Men Are Unhappy and What We Can Do About It* (2020), Matt Rudd found that many successful men are deeply unhappy because they are being driven by what it feels like to be a real man. In a book review article by Christina Patterson called " Man Down review- why are men unhappy? (Sunday Times, September 20th, 2020), she describes how Rudd calls this cultural trap "the Man Box" and includes having status, being tough, strong, successful, a provider, getting a promotion, being a great Dad, and having a fancy house and car. As they struggle to keep up, they have sleepless nights, which saps energy and affects their performance, their career, and their relationships. They are boxed in and can't find a way out. The repressed man then runs on the chimp and reptile systems, with all the chemicals flushing through them, just to help them survive life. The consequence of being driven by false expectations, values and drivers is physical, mental, emotional, and social overload.

When you are unconsciously ashamed of failure, or other unrealistic values drive you to continue, overload happens. When you review the PIES overload, how much were you propelled by values, expectations and norms that don't serve you? The problem is not the values per se, but rather it is not being able to *revise* the values. Loyalty in a healthy relationship at home or at work is a great value to have. But what happens if the workplace or a partner is harming you or putting unrealistic pressures on you? Do you stay loyal and committed? Sometimes loyalty gets you stuck in harsh environments, and it is better to bail out. Likewise, valuing success is great, but not at the cost of health. Valuing health has to take priority.

Have you been "boxed in" by cultural norms and affected by how society is "meant" to function? Did you have unrealistic, unhealthy attitudes and values unconsciously embedded in you, not just about work, but how you should be and how you should care for or provide for others? Take time to review how flexible you are when life becomes unreasonable. Work and lifestyle must be sustainable and achievable long term. Be a mindful independent thinker, stay clear headed and work out what is a balanced lifestyle.

Overload is not just for high-fliers and optimisers and is certainly not exclusive to people who develop CFS and Long Covid. Overload cuts across the whole socio-economic spectrum as ordinary, hardworking people are inundated with chores, lists, financial pressures, and daily hassles, as well as relationship or family demands. Poverty is highly correlated to ill health because living in poverty is arduous. Financial strains impact on our mental, social, and emotional load and can contribute to greater discord or repression, which then further impacts on our emotional, social and mental load. Furthermore, caring for others adds to our physical load; interestingly, it is often the carers who become ill. As pressures come from all directions, it is easy to see how the modern world is awash with conditions affecting the gut, immune system, cardio system, and our susceptibility to infections. The result is also a perfect storm for people getting post viral fatigue, CFS or Long Covid as they tip over into exhaustion, fatigue, and shutdown.

Do a reality check. Is your environment healthy? Is what you are doing healthy? Do you need to let go of certain values and beliefs sometimes, and do what's healthy instead? It isn't true that you have "got to" do everything on your list, certainly not to your optimum level. What are you going to ditch, delegate and do less of? Something has to give, and it cannot be your body.

Other examples of physical overload include:

Sleep Deprivation. There is a high correlation between sleep deprivation and autonomic dysfunction. Furthermore, Harvey Moldofsky (1993) showed that patients with fibromyalgia and chronic fatigue syndrome had abnormal EEG patterns in non-REM sleep, the sleep when muscle and tissue restoration is thought to occur. He goes on to provide evidence that sleep deprivation has "been shown to induce many of the behavioral and somatic features identified in patients with fibromyalgia and chronic fatigue syndrome" (p. 265). This is hardly surprising, as a key function of sleep is to restore the body, to replenish the reserves and to heal the body; hence why it is called restorative sleep. When you look back, did you notice that you had a lack of healthy, restorative sleep before crashing? Were you keeping going for far too many hours, burning the midnight oil to get all your jobs done, squeezing in socialising, and then going to bed with a list of things you still had to do? Were you waking in the middle of the night trying to resolve problems of the day and not getting back to sleep? Burning the candle at both ends socially?

Many conditions are related to poor sleep patterns including cancer, so now you are recovered, do ensure you get into healthy sleeping habits. Were you in the habit of keeping going, without relaxing? The Millennial generation say they don't know how to relax, and this is true of so many people. Physical overload will happen when the body doesn't get enough downtime. We will learn the Art of Relaxation, of simply doing nothing. Develop a consistent sleep routine to reset the circadian cycle.

Viruses and other infections. Moldosky (1993) provides evidence to show there is "a reciprocal relationship of the immune and sleep-wake systems" (p.262). As McEwan said, "when a healthy person is subject to overload, they become susceptible to viruses." Have you noticed that you have been more susceptible to things, even before getting this virus? A common cold doesn't cause CFS and yet it was the one I crashed with every month, for 10 years before actually ending up with CFS because I had become susceptible. Did you bravely keep going, overloaded by restorative sleep deprivation, so focused on carrying on, that you ignored signs that your body wasn't at its peak? Certainly, viruses and serious infections such as Covid-19, Gastroenteritis, malaria and Glandular Fever can overload us, but consider if there was anything making you susceptible and unable to recover? Viruses can cause inflammation but when the sympathetic system stays on, the healthy anti-inflammatory system is off, compounding the problem. In Long Covid, the symptoms will persist when the body's protective system stays on, increasing inflammation. This concurs with Naviaux (2020 p.41) showing at a cellular level, we get stuck in the sickness loop until the body gets the "all clear" signal that it is safe to heal. Inflammation affects joints and muscles, coughing, fatigue, rashes, and headaches. Consider if your lifestyle, for many years before, could have contributed to overload, compromising your immune system, and then the virus was the straw that broke the camel's back.

Diet. We know that diabetes has rocketed in our country due to an unhealthy intake of sugary food, processed food, and drinks. Diabetics are more susceptible to Covid-19 and diabetes research is looking at how our system becomes so overloaded that it cannot sustain attack from viruses. Likewise, years of alcoholic intake, and more generally an indulgent lifestyle, massively impact on our load. High fat and high refined carbohydrate intake are correlated with increased strain on the body's metabolism and increased sympathetic activity, putting the body into red alert and creating low vagal tone.

Inactivity. All patients are now encouraged to move as soon as possible to activate the vagal system and stop the body going into survival mode. Furthermore, inactivity is a factor in memory and learning dysfunction, causing brain fog, a debilitating symptom of CFS and Long Covid. Were you an active person before getting ill? Certainly, the illness caused immobilisation, increasing brain fog and tipping the hypothalamus-pituitary-adrenal axis out of balance (HPA).

I in PIES stands for Intellectual Overload

Physical overload, especially sleep deprivation, can contribute to a mental overload. Behind tasks and chores are decisions, storing and remembering, problem solving, prioritising, negotiations and dealing with setbacks. Emma, a French feminist cartoonist refers to the "mental load" when the household project manager is responsible for a hundred chores. It is this mental load which produces overload because we must consciously remember them, and conscious effort requires huge amounts of energy from the body.

Before you took ill, how much was going on in your head? Was it filled with problems, To Do Lists, resolving problems, and managing your family members' lives as well as your own? Dealing with problems is stimulating and really satisfying; it is when the problems are too big, too many or persist that burden develops. Try juggling thirty balls in reality and see what happens. It is all about reasonable load and balance. Were your problems too big, were there too many conundrums to deal with all at once? Was there an ongoing problem, or insurmountable demands such as a bullying boss, occupying your mind?

Many people don't get out of a job that is adversely affecting them because they just can't find time or energy to add to their to-do list. Likewise, it takes energy, mental resilience, and clarity to go through a relationship break-up. When we are already overloaded, taking on more load is too much, and so people stay in situations that are not healthy and then hit breaking point and wonder why they are ill or developed intolerances. Overload means demands outweigh supply, and your ability to think straight is reduced, so you end up making unhealthy decisions that add to the load.

Mental load is more exhausting than physical hard work. How many people have wondered how we are going to get everything done in time and end up having "errand paralysis" or sleepless nights? The more mental load we have, the less sleep we get and so the less resourceful we are, thus making our physical load more demanding. A downward spiral ensues. It is not just men trapped in the "man box" who suffer this; it is becoming a cultural norm in Western society.

E in PIES stands for Emotional Load

Can you truly identify emotions? When I have done exercises with groups of men and women together, women generally are excellent at identifying what each emotion is and can recognise the feeling of individual emotions; hurt, shame, guilt, anger. Women of course can ignore signs as well or haven't got the time to deal with them. Those on the Autistic Spectrum particularly struggle and load leaks out in somatic ways, from experiencing headaches, tummy upsets, illness and fatigue. In the past 10 years I have been aware that several female clients had been undiagnosed on the autistic spectrum or attention deficit spectrum. Their lives improved dramatically when they got a diagnosis and were taught strategies to prevent overload, particularly social overload because they struggle with the nuances of interaction.

Many men I have worked with cannot easily recognise emotional responses or identify them. This doesn't mean men don't have emotional responses; studies have shown that men actually have a more powerful physiological response than women; they just can't recognise it or express it. Men have been socialised to "man up" to get on with it and are unhealthily taught that being emotional is not manly. This works well, often, but is flawed; if you can't recognise that your own physiology is reacting to a situation, problems can carry on unresolved and often lead to numerous physical, medical and mental issues. Did your early environment enable emotional literacy, enabling you to understand and express emotions, or were you just meant to not make a scene and get on with it? Many men prefer to be active and not talk about things. 2-year-old girls tend to have a greater capacity for expression and language than 2-year-old boys; whilst active skills are necessary and wonderful, some men may be disadvantaged in being unable to verbalise emotions.

Emotions are chemical molecules that adhere to receptors in your body and physically affect your body for good or ill. As humans, we develop the emotional brain before we have cognition, so babies only have emotional responses to everything. We are physically wired, early on, to respond emotionally to every situation; it is part of what it is to be human. The cognitive brain, that has a chance of overriding the emotional brain, only develops - with support - at about four years old. Even as adults, the emotional reaction happens first and then we consciously decide if we need to stop the emotional response and move on. This is the human condition and how the brain works; temperament and early shaping will influence your emotional load and ability to self-regulate and manage emotions healthily.

The diagram on PIES outlines some of the main categories. Have a think - what triggers you to have emotional responses? Here are just some ideas:

Compliance. These people tend to do as they are told and feel guilt, shame, and anxiety when they don't measure up to their own or others' expectations of them. Moral development teaches us to have an internal compass and feel ashamed if we do something morally wrong, rather than rely on a policeman or external force to keep us in check. This is clearly essential for a healthy society but unfortunately, highly conscientious children can then feel bad if they do anything wrong, assuming it must be their fault. This can translate into expressions of low self-esteem, self-loathing, self-blame, and shame. Indeed, many people internalise everything as being "their fault". Critically, they will try harder to get everything right to avoid criticism and feeling bad. This of course increases the physical and mental load as they endeavour to get things right (and keep out of trouble).

Conflict and anger. Many people with CFS will do anything to avoid conflict because it makes them feel physically shaken. It is often easier to do everything yourself than ask for help and create disharmony.

Again, this increases physical and mental load and leads to unbalanced social interactions.

Grief. The death of a loved one has an enormous and lasting impact on our health and mortality. When we lose someone, through death or separation, it can also impact on financial burdens, physical overload and on other relationships. In our culture, we are expected to carry on as normal when going through grief, either because of relationship breakdowns or death. Again, keeping going on only one or two cylinders is like walking on a broken leg.

Bullying. Bullying destroys our self-esteem and performance. The famous "Brown Eyed, Blue Eyed Experiment" carried out by the teacher Jane Elliott in 1968 demonstrates how quickly our academic ability and self-worth are destroyed by bullying, criticism and prejudice. The experiment was originally carried out with children after Martin Luther King was killed but has been replicated with adults and had the same horrifying results. Under current guidelines, this experiment is deemed highly unethical, but it illustrates how emotional overload severely impacts on well-being and performance. There is a link in the reference section and I would recommend watching the power of bullying and victimisation.

Fear and anxiety. The illness itself can trigger fearful, desperate emotions, and these emotions get us stuck in survival mode when they carry on too long. It is normal to have an emotional response to something so terrifying and disabling, but it is essential to let go of it, and to resolve problems or get rid of them.

Before you took ill, even if it was years before, did you notice that you were emotionally overloaded by things and certain people in your environment, affecting your self-esteem or ability to feel relaxed? Emotional overload should not be underestimated because emotions are chemical molecules, attaching to receptors all over our bodies, including the gut, the heart, the immune cells. Healthy emotions heal the organs while distress or stress emotions damage them.

Molecules of emotion affect the whole body, reduce our threshold, increase sleep deprivation, and make demands harder. Adrenals kick in when demands outweigh supply and a vicious cycle develops. For further insights, read *Molecules of Emotion* (1997) by the neuroscientist Candice Pert, and any books by Dr. David Hamilton, a research chemist, including *How the Mind Heals the Body* (2008) and *It's the Thought That Counts* (2008). Also read any research online from the Heartmath Institute, Colorado, which shows how emotions impact on the heart. You do not have to express emotions for them to have an impact on the body. Indeed, repressing emotions has a greater impact.

S in PIES stands for Social Load

Different environments shape us, as this poem by Dorothy Law Nolte illustrates.

"Children Learn What They Live" by Dorothy Law Nolte, Ph.D.

"If children live with criticism, they learn to condemn.
If children live with hostility, they learn to fight.
If children live with fear, they learn to be apprehensive.
If children live with pity, they learn to feel sorry for themselves.
If children live with ridicule, they learn to feel shy.
If children live with jealousy, they learn to feel envy.
If children live with shame, they learn to feel guilty.
If children live with encouragement, they learn confidence.
If children live with tolerance, they learn patience.
If children live with praise, they learn appreciation.
If children live with acceptance, they learn to love.
If children live with approval, they learn to like themselves.
If children live with recognition, they learn it is good to have a goal.
If children live with sharing, they learn generosity.
If children live with honesty, they learn truthfulness.
If children live with fairness, they learn justice.
If children live with kindness and consideration, they learn respect.
If children live with security, they learn to have faith in
themselves and in those about them.
If children live with friendliness, they learn the world
is a nice place in which to live."

How were you treated in the early years? Clearly, the outcomes aren't always the same for every child; for instance, a child who lives with criticism and disapproval is just as likely to develop low self-esteem, self-loathing, shame, and a lack of confidence in themselves, affecting performance and their response to life.

Your early years environment has a profound effect on development because it is at this age the brain is shaped and it is making sense of the world. Tragically, in the UK, there are a million children brought up with abuse or domestic violence, which has lifelong consequences unless worked through. Many others have lived with shouting, disapproval and put downs. The Jesuit saying, "give me a boy until he is seven, and I will show you the man" has some truth, because 80% of how we are formed is in those early years. These children then have to try harder than others to do life easily; lacking the fundamental building blocks decreases supply, robustness, and therefore increases load.

We are biologically programmed to go into arousal when exposed to a harsh tone of voice and facial expression. Remember, another person's tone of voice and facial expression physically changes your breathing and heartbeat (Porges 2011 p.13). A child who experienced this early on in life, whether it was anger, criticism, non-attachment, or emotional blackmail, feels highly aroused on the inside but has no outlet to express it. An angry voice embeds fear, while criticism embeds shame and low self-esteem. I have worked with so many men who have achieved great things, pushed themselves to the limit, and yet still feel uneasy and incomplete. They were, metaphorically, doing triple back somersaults, unconsciously waiting in vain for the day their Dad said, "I'm proud of you", and getting ill or exhausted in the process. As one man said, "If I won gold at the Olympics, my Dad would still think it wasn't good enough; I should have won two. His voice became my critical self-talk." No wonder they got trapped in the Man Box that Rudd describes.

Every loving parent gets angry and can be critical, but this is not the same as living with it constantly. As research by McEwan, Porges and Sapolsky point out, it is the chronic, long-term exposure that leads to chronic fatigue and other illnesses. It is not fair that a child grows up with such emotional load, affecting performance, but it certainly isn't uncommon. We can become great friends with the critical parent later in life, but the shaping remains, unless we consciously change it and stop the automatic reaction to triggers.

Was there anything in your environment growing up that would have affected your emotional overload and is then triggered even in adulthood? Are you prickly, defensive, or put down by anything that isn't dulcet tones and approval? Once we have become conditioned to respond in a certain way to a trigger, we will respond like this forever, unless we are taught to consciously change it. The trigger is often other people's role, tone of voice or facial expression.

Consider whether your environment now, or in the past was entirely nurturing, enabling you to thrive. Was there anything or anyone triggering physical, mental, emotional, and social overload? Organisms adapt to survive harsh conditions. What type of environment shaped you? What environment did you live in before becoming ill? You will struggle to recover and stay healthy if you are still living in unfavourable environments because we need healthy conditions and secure, loving support to thrive as adults.

As social animals, we are created to be part of a pack and to have social interaction with others. Professor Julianne Holt-Lunstad (2010) carried out a meta-analysis, examining 148 studies that explored the major causes of death in humans. Lack of a social network ranked as highest risk, above a poor diet, lack of exercise, and exposure to pollution. So friendships and having another person to confide in are really important buffers against life's hurdles. Also, Robert Dunbar (2021), an eminent anthropologist, primate behaviourist and psychologist, carried out a large-scale analysis across Europe, and found that five close friends is optimal for avoiding depression. Today, researchers are able to measure how our bodies respond at a cellular level, creating sickness behaviour such as head, muscle and abdominal aches, changes in the gut microbiome, and sleep deprivation and fatigue due to diverse threats. Naviaux (2020 p. 45) cites the findings of Eric Shattuck and Michael Muehlenbein,(2015) showing, "these threats can be as diverse as an infection, poisoning, physical, or psychological trauma, and still trigger the *same* stereotyped sickness behaviour"). Our social environment impacts on the body as much as any other physical threat; social connections act as buffers against life's stresses and strains, balancing out overload. Have you had sustained periods of isolation or lack of support from significant others? Certainly, the illness can impact hugely on social deprivation because many people spend most of their time isolated and lose friends.

However, sometimes, rather than having a lack of social support, social interaction can be too much. A large social network, or others being dependent on you, by definition, increases physical tasks and mental load, as there are only so many hours in a day to fit everything in. Pressures can then create emotional arousal and the body has no down time to recover. It is the balance that matters; did it feel easy or were you spinning too many plates? Burning the candle at both ends for fear of missing out? Can you say no to people when you know that taking on more is unhealthy?

Social anxiety is common in our society, partly because in terms of evolution, being isolated or rejected is unhealthy; humans survive better in a pack with their tribe. Comparison and self-consciousness can lower self-esteem and competence; when resourcefulness is lowered, the gap between supply and demand increases and so the survival Autonomic Nervous System is constantly activated.

Societal and cultural pressures, errand paralysis, and a need to conform to unrealistic expectations massively influence PIES overload. Before you took ill or previously, was there conflict, societal pressures, or discord in your life? Was there a significant person who abandoned or rejected you, affecting your core trust, competency, and attachments, meaning you need to try harder to achieve? Was your environment nurturing and balanced?

Overload of an Extreme Kind

Many people who had chronic fatigue syndrome (CFS), or Long Covid, lived in healthy conditions prior to becoming ill and just needed to learn how to get out of the perpetual sickness loop and fatigue from a virus or infection. Others had a healthy life but had a particular time in life when they were unreasonably overloaded with PIES, and they returned to healthy conditions once recovered. However, many clients also lived in extreme circumstances, prior to the illness, so check if any of the following resonates with you:

Dysfunctional Relationships. A dysfunctional relationship is when it isn't working for one or both people. There will be some imbalance of power, control, needs and care. A nurturing relationship will have discord and disharmony sometimes, but essentially it will feel healthy. A dysfunctional relationship will feel hard and unnurturing - it can appear wonderful, as long as the person holding the power is happy and accommodated.

Coercive Abuse. If you are in a relationship that involves coercive abuse, then it is going to be very hard for you to recover and stay healthy. Coercion is when one person holds distorted power through control, possessiveness, anger, and put-downs. There are definite signs of coercion, according to Cali Estes, a clinical psychologist. This is a list of pointers from her and from victims' experiences:

- They isolate you from friends and family, and often want you to move from a place where you had established friends and who would have offered a clear perspective on your relationship.
- They monitor your everyday life, such as phoning to find out where you are, and restricting you to when you should be home and checking calls. They want to know where you have been and why.
- They deny you freedom and restrict access to others and activities. If you are "allowed" to go to work because the household needs your income, you must be home at a designated time, or else.
- They wear you down and convince you that you are wrong, telling you repeatedly you are not a good enough, committed partner. They often get angry if anything isn't exactly how they want it and how they want you to be.
- In isolation, hearing only their voice, you become unsure of what is normal and try harder to get it right for the perpetrator, to keep the peace.
- They will do put-downs to keep you in your place and gain control, destroy your confidence and weaken you. They call you selfish if you aren't entirely focused on them, or lazy if you don't have everything perfect when they arrive home.
- In different gender relationships, the man will want the woman to be the homemaker and child carer, and they are threatened if her work role and income are more than his. She does all the roles, even if she works full time; otherwise, she is constantly

told she is a bad wife, housekeeper, and mother. They won't help you because you don't give them what they need: control, exclusive love, adoration, and attention.

- They need sexual attention, often daily. Any rejection or lack of enthusiasm leads to payback.
- They will try to turn the children against you and get them on their side, especially when they start to feel like they are losing control.

Whilst men are the perpetrators 95% of the time (Merseyside Domestic Abuse data, Barlow 2018) it can also be women who control and victimise. I have worked with several men who endured awful relationships and have been too frightened to separate and risk leaving the children with her. Anyone living with a parent, or other person, with a personality disorder or narcissistic traits will be affected and struggle to survive, unless they seek help.

Coercive abuse has only been recognised as an illegal practice in the UK since 2015 but even now, few perpetrators are prosecuted, and few women go forward. The latest available estimates from the Crime Survey for England and Wales (CSEW) showed that over four in five victims (83%) of partner abuse did not report the abuse to the police. The report says CSEW estimates do not completely capture the new offence of coercive and controlling behaviour. New survey questions to better estimate experiences of this type of abuse are still under development (ONS 2018). Before 2015, coercion was considered a private matter within a marriage, no matter how difficult the situation. Until as recently as 1969, it was illegal for women to divorce, unless she could prove adultery, drunkenness, desertion, rape, or physical cruelty. Often people stay in unhealthy relationships for many reasons. Coercion is still not recognised in the USA, unless a crime has been committed. Bizarrely, it is legal to abuse another person mentally, emotionally, and socially, but not to damage property in the process!

Being in one of these relationships has nothing to do with being stupid or pathetic; very successful, intelligent, kind, healthy men and women can get embroiled with a controlling partner because, in the beginning, it is wonderful and there are few early warning signs. We can be academically brilliant but didn't learn healthy relationships growing up. According to research into the cycle of abuse, there is a definite pattern:

- Stage one is the honeymoon period, the forming stage of being on our best behaviour. As with normal relationships, you want to spend lots of time together, and they are charming and committed. You accommodate each other's quirks and have rose coloured glasses on.
- Stage two of any healthy relationship is when the honeymoon period is over, and life returns to normal, dividing attention between work, chores, family, and friends. In all healthy relationships, this is when differences and compromises need to be worked through and there will be disagreements before compromises are negotiated. Now the real problems start. They still want the exclusive "truly, madly, deeply" stage of love, and see your divided attention as a rebuff to this. They want to be with you everywhere you go, and when you say you need some space or time to do other things, they may try to accommodate, but it never lasts. At this stage you may have endless talks as you try to reason and reassure them.
- The third stage is abusive control. In a healthy relationship, you go through the honeymoon stage, you find a healthy balance, and compromise on a variety of issues, so both parties have their needs met and you develop a balanced, healthy relationship, give and take. This is when coercion becomes obvious. Control is their only way to feel secure and empowered. As they feel they are losing control and attention, unrealistic demands increase, they get angrier, and increase their control over all aspects of your life. They will humiliate you, put you down, and belittle you. They will isolate you from friends and family through control, jealousy, and a conviction that friends or family will turn you against him. They tend to have a rigid personality, where things are black and white, and they have a fixed idea how things "should be", including the house, children, work hours, what you wear and your level of social contact. There will be payback if you don't measure up; everything is a reflection on how much you love and respect them. Sadly, having fallen off the pedestal, you fall short all the time, forever failing. They thrive on making up after conflict, as it makes them feel loved, just like in the honeymoon period.

Recovery isn't enough. You must determine to find a more nurturing environment for yourself. As Kiecolt-Glaser and Glaser (1991) found in their research, marital strife has a greater impact on health than physical burden, or any other type of stress. Please contact a counsellor. Do get support urgently and get advice from Citizens Advice about your financial and physical circumstances. Your mental and physical health was destroyed by years of abuse constantly activating the stress response, no matter how bravely you tried to keep going. It is not an environment where you can thrive, and you will be lucky to survive. Relate Counselling will see clients individually and you only donate whatever you feel you can afford. Do not worry about the people who don't understand.

Accommodating Others When It Is Unhealthy. Accommodating others, in itself, is a normal, healthy trait. In any healthy relationship, we accommodate each other, make allowances, make things nice for them, but it is reciprocal. It comes from love, compromise, teamwork and merging as a couple. Each has their needs and interests met, as much as it is reasonable, and they are okay to compromise. We accommodate our children all the time, and that is part of nurturing, just as they will learn empathy, to give and take, and to share and to consider others.

However, accommodating others when it isn't reciprocal, through fear, or to keep the peace, is a dysfunctional relationship and an unhealthy environment to live in. You can't thrive and live in the healthy parasympathetic mode when there are so many triggers. There are many types of dysfunctional relationships that could make your environment hard to live in, but essentially it will start to feel hard, and exhausting. It will start to dawn that your needs aren't being met but their needs are. A relationship should be nurturing, two ways, despite the niggles. You can come to feel it is normal as every relationship establishes norms within it, but the body holds the score as you try harder and harder to make everything happy and harmonious.

Did you have someone who had to be accommodated in your early years environment? Fawning is the fourth survival instinct, when we are powerless. Not everyone accommodates; your siblings' strategy may have been to fight or flight against the dysfunctional powerhouse. Maybe you were in that situation before being ill? Think, what would happen if you said no to them, or didn't go along with them? What if you demanded to have your needs and desires met? Would they scream, shout, walk out or reject you?

Do they consider and accommodate your needs and plans? If you live with or lived with someone like this, there is a good chance you became overloaded and hit the threshold through emotional load, mental load (always calculating how to keep everything happy) and physical load, as you take the pressure off them.

Life on the surface often seems very happy and devoid of conflict but if the harmony comes at the cost of overload, health and not having one's own needs met, then it is peace and happy families, at a price.

The Tipping Point for Chronic Fatigue Syndrome and Related Illnesses

Did it feel like everything was okay and the illness appeared to come "out of the blue"? Or were the PIES building up a long time before the crash? Illness may have been purely due to a powerful virus like Covid-19, but consider if there were other factors in play? The tipping point can happen over many years, or since childhood.

The Catastrophe Theory diagram below demonstrates how the load eventually reached critical mass and tipped the scales. Catastrophe theory, a mathematical model, applies to so many aspects of nature and illnesses. Volcanoes and earthquakes didn't suddenly happen; there was a build-up under the surface. Likewise, CFS, cancer and other health conditions build up. It is worth considering if you could have been functioning at peak performance, hovering around the maximum healthy threshold, and with few reserves left in the tank, which made you more susceptible to infections or less able to fight them.

Diagram of Catastrophe Theory and Sudden Tipping Point

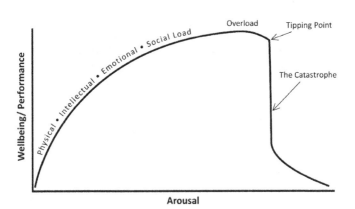

It is empowering to know that changing or removing environmental factors can reduce load and restore health. You may need to just tweak a few things or you may need to make bigger changes, but you will do *whatever* it takes to be healthy.

Reflecting on Overload and How to Reduce It

Have a Clear Perception. A part of overload is the belief that you have no other choice, and that you have got to keep going. When overloaded, you haven't got time to think clearly; you are in autopilot, just existing. If you were relying on the chimp and rocket fuels to keep going, your thinking will be reactive, not rational. Take time to quietly reflect on how you want to do life and notice any limiting beliefs, then commit to stopping them, and use the Traffic Light approach to access clear-headedness.

Here is a true story from a previous 27-year-old client of mine named Annabelle, who recovered from CFS some years ago. She contacted me to say she was feeling overwhelmed:

> "I *am doing really well physically but becoming more anxious, worrying about the future, and anticipating*

disaster. I feel like I should have my own house by now, I should be getting a promotion, have a steady job, and settling down like my parents did, and it is too much. My mind is always racing, thinking about what I need to do and how I am going to cope, and it just feels impossible. In all honesty it's overwhelming and has become an all-consuming part of my life that I should be doing life better, following a certain path. I'm always just catching up and never feel that I am achieving. Adulting is so hard, and I don't feel like an adult. This is affecting my relationships; I recently backed off from my five-year relationship as I feel like there is too much pressure to be ready to settle."

We talked about how her generation needed to establish new healthy beliefs and realistic expectations about what is achievable and relevant to the world they live in. It is unhelpful to try being like previous generations who had very different opportunities and drivers. She agreed that meeting unrealistic goals was unhealthy. Annabelle had been driven by a need to get promotion, and to provide a better income for "adulting". This led to physical, emotional, and mental overload. Changing her perception enabled her to get off the treadmill, stop, and think clearly about what really matters.

She enjoyed her work and had supportive colleagues, a great partner, lovely friends and could afford to live on the current income. She could meet friends for coffee instead of eating out, and decided renting a flat was fine. When she was no longer anxious about having to get a house and promotion, she realised a load had been taken off her. Crucially, she spoke to someone about the problem and gave herself time to solve the problem instead of keeping going.

Think how you need to revise beliefs, values, and expectations. Spend time reviewing how to take the load off and give your brain a well-earned rest. Don't conform to society and cultural environmental norms; be an independent thinker. What is right for you to stay healthy?

Maybe the job that you once loved and found stimulating has changed dramatically and is now too challenging or exhausting but you are still pushing on. Find time to have a healthier life.

Kate's story

"I started off loving my job as a primary school teacher but doing a 12-hour day and working weekends was draining on top of all the other chores. My head was full of stuff, I had gut problems, I kept getting respiratory infections and was tired all the time. I was literally just putting one foot in front of the other. It was really frightening to think of letting go of a secure job, with great colleagues and taking a leap of faith into the unknown but to find a healthier lifestyle, I had to take a chance, set aside the fear, and focus on possibilities, not on obstacles. I had to find time to search, do application forms and revise my CV. I knew if I didn't, I would get stuck forever and go under.

I am so glad I took the leap and jumped off the treadmill. I have a job now, where I work 9-5, with evenings and weekends off. I have a balanced life and it's amazing how much healthier I am working in a healthy work environment. I'm no longer tired all the time; my gut is better, and I am less prone to respiratory infections. I am so happy I had the courage to get out."

Kate was very brave to make the move and wise to take time out to review her life. Likewise, whatever you value, give it your time; don't just struggle on. Have you lost sight of possibilities, that there could be another way? Humans are born explorers; somewhere in the middle of adulting, some people stop being excited by possibilities and become cautious and concerned about providing and managing their daily responsibilities. The day my daughters said, "we don't care if we live in a caravan, as long as you are healthy", was the day I was free; free to let go of all the mental overload that had been affecting recovery, free to become self-employed and take a risk.

When you remove yourself from unhealthy environments and unhealthy norms, your body adapts and lives in the healthy mode, just like Kate, when she actively found better working conditions. There is no substitute for a healthy environment. If you get stuck in a loop, always finding reasons not to make changes, then maybe you need a coach, an NLP practitioner, or a best friend to give you a nudge. Check out if that is a pattern of yours. Annabelle only needed 30 minutes to change her perception of life and improve wellbeing. Stop the chimp running the show. Be FEARLESS.

Life Balance. Adulting isn't meant to be just about chores, targets, and responsibilities. Remember as a teenager how much you wanted to be a grown up because grown-ups can make choices? When you are fully recovered, check that you have got the life balance right, being FEARLESS.

Exercise. Spend a month colour-coding your life. Have a colour for WORK / RESPONSIBILITIES, and another colour for REST / SLEEP. Use an additional colour for LEISURE / RELAX / ENJOYMENT.

Check out if you have a balance, and if not, why? Are you living in autopilot rather than living consciously? Change requires time-out to reflect and gain clarity. If you don't have time to colour code, then you definitely haven't got a work-life balance!

The body thrives when it is doing things it loves, and it barely survives when it isn't. At the moment, work out what you can do to get a healthy work-life balance, and what needs to go. You can coach yourself but if you employ a mentor, a buddy, or a coach, you have a greater chance of breaking habits and succeeding. Make time to relax and enjoy life; prioritise and ditch anything that isn't essential. Focus on what you want, not on what you don't want.

Improved Sleep. Go back and review the section on sleep in BETTER exercises as sleep deprivation is highly correlated to many illnesses, including CFS. Commit to spending time developing healthier sleep routines and better restorative sleep. Sleep is essential for healthy living and your body prefers routines, so make it a priority to establish a sleep pattern. When the circadian cycle is out of sync, the body goes out of sync. Get back to nature, how you are biologically programmed to live, by sleeping when it is dark and rising when it is light. Go outdoors in a full moon if you can. Go camping for a week to reset the body that has been affected by unnatural light and blue light from computer or mobile phone screens. If light isn't natural, the body has probably not fully adapted to it and artificial light enables us to keep going when the body is designed to stop. Sleep between 11 pm and 3 pm detoxes the body, so get into a pattern of being asleep by 11pm. Sleep is the body's natural healer and restores functions in the body. Prioritise sleep over everything.

Viruses. Most people trivialise viruses and return to normal activities when they are not fully fit, expending energy that is meant for fighting infection. This in turns makes them more susceptible to viruses and less able to fight off the infection. Rest, and do the work already outlined, to recover. You are meant to have low energy when the mitochondria are diverting supplies to fight infection.

If you have developed recurrent post-viral fatigue, then either your response to infections or your lifestyle is unhealthy and unreasonable. Prioritise your health. GPs have little time to go back through your records, so it is imperative you flag up your background to your GP, especially if your GP doesn't know you well. When I was diagnosed with CFS, my GP went back through my records, and was shocked to discover that I had had post viral fatigue after every bout of the common cold for 10 years. I hadn't given myself time to fully recover because it felt like I just had to keep going, then succumbed again.

After a bad experience, many people with post viral fatigue syndrome (PVFS) or Long Covid become conditioned to associate "getting a virus" with "having fatigue again". This is completely unconscious. Your protective brain has hardwired viruses to mean threat, and that will automatically turn on the survival system, our pesky chimp and reptile. You had a bad experience but that does not mean it will happen again. In future, consciously recognise that a virus is just a virus; it does not mean you are going to have Long Covid, post viral fatigue or CFS again. Consciously, deliberately, dissociate viruses from fatigue or CFS. Retrain the amygdala to register viruses as something you can overcome. Stay calm, confident and know you will recover. Do seek assistance from a practitioner if you, understandably, find it tricky to do the journey to recovery purely on your own. Much of my follow-up support is preventing meltdowns and extended illness when clients get viruses back. Even years later, if I haven't recovered in a few days, alarm bells ring and I need to practise what I preach. I learnt to voice the fear so others could reassure me when I had a wobble.

When you next get a virus, review the recovery strategies from chapters three to six and be completely confident that you will recover.

Use your Traffic Lights to access all the different FEARLESS resources you need for recovery. FEARLESS won't get you up and running if you are still fighting a virus but it will stop you getting stuck. You may have been subpar before getting a virus, so check out if there was any overload that could have contributed to it. If you are an enthusiast, become aware that we need good reserves to deal with the unexpected, including viruses, so don't live at full capacity. Notice if your body had been telling you to take your foot off the throttle.

Use D3 and supplements to Boost the Immune System. Over ten years ago, the leaders of the European Parliament discussed their concerns that 50% of the European population are deficient in Vitamin D. American Journal of Clinical Nutrition). Vitamin D deficiency that is not sufficiently treated is associated with COVID-19 risk. Testing and treatment for vitamin D deficiency to address COVID-19 warrants aggressive pursuit and study (Meltzer et al, 2020). Further research was carried out by Dr Hermann Brenner and Dr Ben Schottker (2020 p.3642). They measured people's interleukin 6 levels, which are the inflammatory cytokines, in hospitalised patients. Hospitalised people had lower Vitamin D3 to those who didn't require hospitalisation. People with low levels of Vitamin D were six times more likely to need a mechanical ventilator and fourteen times more likely to die. They found 9 out of 10 people who die of Covid-19 had Vitamin D3 deficiency. Furthermore, Vitamin D levels are more likely to affect risk than any other factor including age, gender, or comorbidity factors. Vitamin D3 lowers the risk of acute respiratory infection because it is a hormone in the anti- inflammatory healing process.

A great deal of research is now emerging about the impact of the hormone Vitamin D3 on the immune system, specifically on its role in the anti-inflammatory process. The UK Government currently recommends 400 universal units daily, but research is suggesting that 3000 units is needed in Northern Hemispheres during winter months, from October to March. For further reading, go to the Vitamin D Society website (https://www.vitamindsociety.org/).

On an anecdotal level, whilst I have fully recovered from CFS, I continued to be much more affected by the common cold than other people. I had to take to my bed for about 2 days after catching it and used my mindfulness, FEARLESS tools, and Traffic Lights to ensure I didn't sabotage successful recovery. I had to stay completely calm and wait for my body to fully recover, which it always did within a few more days.

However, for the first time in 30 years, having taken Vitamin D3 every day for many months, I caught a cold, and not only did I not have to lie down, but I didn't feel ill and fatigued either. I just carried on as normal with a runny nose and cold! To me, this has been miraculous; maybe I had been deficient in Vitamin D3 and needed a boost to get my immune system functioning properly? I now take 3000 units in the winter and reduce to 1000 units from March to October, which is what is being recommended by many scientists. See what effect Vitamin D3 has on you and your body's response to viruses.

Healthy Social Environment. In the next chapter we look at how people with CFS may not have learnt the essential defence skills needed to remain robust. When these skills are missing, social interaction, unless it is easy and friendly, can feel challenging and cause overload. It would be useful for you to consider just how much social interaction you need to be healthy.

Actively start to surround yourself with people who nurture you and spend less time, if any, with people who don't. Most people only need to tweak a few things about their environment. Others need to make big changes; I lost a husband but gained permanent health and well-being.

Reducing Emotional Overload. Some people deal with a lot more heartache, conflict, or grief in life because not everyone has the same life. If you have suffered grief and loss, then it is a good idea to access as much support and professional counselling as possible. As a rule of thumb, if grief isn't resolved within two years, you may need assistance to move on. Eye Movement Desensitisation and Reprocessing (EMDR) Therapy is excellent for dealing with any shock or trauma. Likewise, if you live with any unhealthy relationship, it is essential to access support from Relate or any service specialising in this.

Many people have emotions suppressed for many reasons, but physical leakage may suggest all is not well; you start to notice if you get headaches, gut reaction, back tension, fatigue, in response to emotional load. In the next chapter we will do Traffic Lights to choose how to respond better.

Our stiff upper lip culture means we just keep going and present to the world as best we can, which is actually a great thing. It means we become resilient, strong and help ourselves. However, it is not useful if you are putting on a brave face but missing fundamental blocks needed to navigate life better. The majority of clients with CFS or Long Covid needed to learn how to tweak environmental conditions, then carried on being fully healthy. However, a number of people cannot move forward until traumas or scars have been resolved. There is no shame in this; no child chooses to live with abuse, control, neglect or abandonment and the effects they leave, but you can choose to take responsibility and do whatever it takes to break free from the shackles of any past influencer. Any single shock can stir the reptile, making us freeze, and this pattern remains *until* we consciously resolve it. Today, research recognises the impact of transition on children, affecting their academic, social, and emotional development. Consequently, all schools now have transition programmes for every pupil moving to secondary school. Again, EMDR has the best outcome to get people back on track, no matter how many years later.

Access Further Support. As mentioned before, you need to ensure you are functioning in the parasympathetic system before taking expensive supplements, because it is this system which enables digestion and absorption.

If symptoms persist, after mastering everything in the book, you may need to engage further expertise from a GP, a dietician, a nutritionist, or immunologist. There can be other conditions running alongside CFS or PVFS that need to be addressed, or there could be an undiagnosed issue. Of the many hundreds of clients I have worked with, I have only ever met three clients who had done the work consistently and correctly, and then we realised that there was something else going on for them. After further investigation, one lady was diagnosed with a heart condition and two clients had undiagnosed autoimmune disease.

The GP will do a range of tests and refer for others, if need be, based on initial tests. Tests will rule out anaemia, vitamin B12 deficiency, infection or inflammation, kidney, liver, thyroid problems, and diabetes. Some people feel the NHS does not offer sensitive enough tests for thyroid, but it will show if you are in the normal range. You can pay privately to request further thyroid tests. Here are some examples of conditions that can cause similar symptoms to CFS:

- If you have joint pain, you will be tested for a range of rheumatic diseases, including polymyalgia, and blood tests should alert GPs to rarer autoimmune diseases.
- Some gastrointestinal diseases may cause fatigue but are almost always accompanied with diarrhoea or weight loss.
- Hormonal conditions can lead to fatigue, so blood and urine tests can help detect this. For instance, Addison's disease causes fatigue.
- Infections from Lyme disease, viral hepatitis, glandular fever (Epstein Barr virus) and Q fever trigger fatigue.
- Severe sleep conditions, like sleep apnoea will create fatigue and is diagnosed by having sleep measured overnight.

EXERCISE. Draw your diagram of the PIES flower. In each section, add everything that increases a load on you. Include any overload prior to the illnesses, and any cumulative load built up over years.

Healthy PIES - Healthy Load. Now do another flower diagram. Add in any healthy environmental factors you can think of, from nurturing people, healthy relationships, reasonable workload, rest, relaxation, and fun.

Pin these on your wall to remind you of overload and healthy living.

Work out what really matters and what you can change. You will be aware by now that saying "I can't" is often a limiting belief and ensures that you are focused on the barriers and not the possibilities. Just start with asking whether you *could* change your job, or do fewer tasks, or spend time investigating better opportunities for yourself.

Health must be your number one focus and priority, because nothing and nobody is ever going to pull you down again and strip you of wellbeing. Become mindful of your situation and more aware of how your environment impacts on health.

Summary

- It is always better to live in a healthy environment, because all organisms thrive in healthy environments and struggle to survive in unfavourable environments. This is the General Adaptive Syndrome (GAS) borne out by modern research.

- CFS was created when a healthy normal body sustained a long period of chronic overload, or, it could have been a period in your life when you were bombarded with all the plates coming at you at one time. An acute trauma or an infection like sepsis, Glandular Fever, Covid-19 or malaria can also trigger the condition.
- Overload could have started in the early years by growing up in a harsh environment or with a particularly imposing individual. If so, the body may have been activated for years.
- We need to ensure our environment is reasonable, realistic for us and not based on unrealistic expectations.
- Consider what was overloading you before you took ill and what is overloading you now. Was it truly only the virus or some other factors?
- Notice that all these parts of the PIES impact on each other, so there is a domino effect. The more mental load, the more you struggle with physical load, and so on. Marital strife and lack of a support network has more impact on health than physical tasks or any other factor.
- Coercive abuse, or any abuse, severely impacts on physical health. Strive for a healthier environment.
- Commit to eliminating as many unnecessary tasks as possible by changing your belief that you must do them.
- Ditch anything non-essential to allow time for fun and investigate new opportunities. Spend time on what matters. Find a coach or practitioner to help you make changes to your employment and lifestyle.
- Review the section on sleep in BETTER exercises. Sleep is crucial for maintaining health.
- Reduce demands so you don't need to rely on the turbo fuel and the survival mechanisms.
- WORK, REST AND PLAY. Find balance in everything.
- If you can't change people or situations that are affecting your health, leave. Find a healthier environment.
- If you live in the Northern Hemisphere, consider taking 3000 units of Vitamin D3 in the winter and 1000 units in summer.
- Dissociate the connection of "viruses mean fatigue" in future. They don't. Rest when you have a virus and do your FEARLESS

and vagal exercises, using the Traffic Lights to stop saboteurs.

- If you feel there may be other deficiencies, once your parasympathetic nervous system is functioning again, consult your GP for tests, a nutritionist, dietician, or immunologist for further investigation and support.

Chapter 8: Staying Healthy: Becoming More Resourceful

*"In the face of strong winds, let me be a blade of grass.
In the face of strong walls, let me be a gale of wind." -
A traditional Quaker saying.*

As McEwan (2002) said, "Even the most finely tuned stress response in the healthiest of individuals can begin to cause damage if activated again and again over a long period. In other words, chronic stress can cause illnesses...including CFS". So why have we been activated again and again? It may be that we were born with a more easily aroused autonomic system. Additional research by Benjamin N. Goertzel and his colleagues came to similar conclusions. "The fact that only 28 out of several million possible (single nucleotide polymorphism) SNPs predict whether a person has CFS with 76% accuracy, indicates that CFS has a genetic component." (Goertzel et al, 2006 p.475)

In further studies, and using genetic programming, Goertzel and colleagues (2006) concluded: "Among CFS patients, but not controls, a high level of allostatic load was significantly associated with lower median values (indicating worse health) of body pain, physical functioning and general symptom frequency/intensity." This work was supported by the work of Elizabeth Maloney and colleagues (2006, p.467), which showed that "CFS was associated with a high level of allostatic load".

This means we may have a predisposition to activate the adaptive system. If you have a biological propensity to turn on the chimp and the reptile, then the risk of developing chronic fatigue syndrome (CFS) is obviously much higher. I personally think that we are born with a more easily activated system. We didn't choose it any more than we choose eye colour. But it could also have been compounded if we were exposed to any form of threatening environment throughout life. Either way, it is not your fault. Maybe the current genetic CFS research will explain why our reptilian system was activated during CFS and Long Covid, whilst other people who are chronically activated get stuck in chimp mode and have other illnesses such as heart disease, gut problems, and strokes.

Sapolsky, in his book *Why Zebras Don't Get Ulcers* (2004), explains that "we differ in how fast our adrenals make glucocorticoids", a majorly important stress chemical. He reviewed research showing that people with "chronic fatigue are in sustained arousal" and have inappropriate levels of stress chemicals. This means there *may* be innate factors and certainly the defence systems stay on for too long during the illness.

If you stop to consider for a moment, have you always been a zebra, reacting momentarily to a situation and reverting to base instantly, or was your physiology affected by things, and stayed on, even after the event had passed? As a child, were you "thick skinned", so nothing affected your physiology, or were you easily aroused internally, especially if hurt by criticism or exposed to anger? I know that even as a little child, I felt physically shaken when I was shouted at. Did you freeze, and become speechless? Did you stand and take it because you were powerless, but felt physically affected internally? Children are rarely allowed to run from a frightening parent or to fight them, so in those circumstances, the reptilian response is all they have, and then it is used habitually over the years. Clearly, freeze mode as a child is a great survival mechanism because it is better to put up with the situation than it is to rile the tiger even more. However, it is not a great strategy for long term health and sustainability. Likewise, activating the chimp early on will become the default mode in any threatening situation.

Social and emotional buffers are our greatest defence;" Social support is getting the system to help regulate our autonomic state." Porges (2015, p.6). This means social support literally calms our physiology and turns on the healthy, healing system whilst an angry face activates the chimp. Apart from taking the load off us, a nurturing tone and facial expressions keep us physically calm and strengthen us; without them we are easily activated. Hence, social isolation and strife are a recipe for ill health.

Babies and toddlers only have instinct to respond to situations, so the tone of voice and faces they are exposed to shapes their physiology and their habitual response to the world. Every loving parent gets angry and can be critical, but this is not the same as living with it constantly. When life is harsh, the child will be shaped differently and therefore respond to the world differently, compared to a child growing up in a nurturing atmosphere. As McEwan, Porges and Sapolsky point out, it is the *chronic*, long-term exposure that leads to chronic fatigue and other illnesses. What was your perception of growing up and which survival mechanism repetitively fired off?

If you have been programmed early on to be vigilant, then you are conditioned to heightened arousal by any sign of criticism, conflict, or discord. If you have an innate tendency to turn on the reptile and have been exposed to threatening expressions at a young age, then the risk of developing a malfunctioning neurological condition is obviously much higher.

We can be brought up in the most loving, supportive, and healthy family and still succumb to CFS illnesses. Certainly, you may have been a "lamb to the slaughter" who was sent into the big wide world as a young adult, and unprepared for meeting people with aggressive or dysfunctional personalities.

In this chapter, we will look at how we increase supply to meet demands by activating our social communicative skills for defence. Even when we live in a healthy environment, surrounded by balanced, supportive people, there will be times when we have to deal with difficult situations and people.

I believe improving defence skills is necessary for the vast majority of people, not just those who develop chronic fatigue syndrome. Other people may not get CFS, but they may develop heart disease, myocarditis, thyroid problems, hypertension, gut problems, strokes, allergies, intolerances, or a myriad of other leakages, because the body holds the score.

Overload may be perceived by some, especially men, to be a weakness and associate weakness with failure or shame. Blame or shame is pointless; we simply need to become more resourceful and stay healthy. This chapter will show you how to skill up, how to react less to your environment, and be the robust person you need to be for recovery and long-term well-being. You can access the online training at www. resettothrive.co.uk, to see exactly how to practise skills that may not have been triggered automatically, in certain situations.

The Missing Piece of the Jigsaw: the Human Social Defence Mode

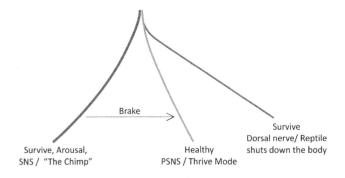

The three branches of the Autonomic Nervous System (ANS)

So, let's look at a seminal piece of work by Stephen Porges (2001 p.123) on Polyvagal Theory that has given us a much better understanding of CFS and other similar conditions. Based on Polyvagal research, in the past few years there has been a wealth of treatments based on vagal activation for a range of conditions, including cardiac, respiratory, gut, and autoimmune.

In his Polyvagal Theory, he identifies three levels of defence for human beings, not just the mammalian chimp defence system and the reptilian defence system, that we have focused on throughout the book. These are:

LEVEL 1: Human Social Engagement Mode. This defence system activates our healthy ventral vagus nerve, the one that enables our body to function and thrive, represented as green on our ANS diagram above. Vagus means wandering and this major nerve is attached to most major organs in the body. It connects to the facial muscles and auditory system to detect tone of voice and expression via the cranial nerve. It is the most recent defence mechanism we have developed as a species, and the one we should be using all the time. Most of the time, other people or situations are not life threatening, so we don't need to go into fight and flight mode; we just need to use our social skills to deal with any discord or conflict. This means we use our facial expression, tone of voice, and expressions to resolve the conflict, which ensures we stay in the calm, healthy parasympathetic system. These are our primary defence mechanisms that should be used *all* the time, unless there is real, potential danger. The healthy vagus nerve also kicks in quickly to put the brakes on the chimp, inhibiting the sympathetic system, when it calibrates that the threat isn't really a big deal.

For example, a neighbour may look raging as he shouts at you because your tree is shading his garden but going into sympathetic chimp mode to deal with his anger is too extreme a reaction and not good for the body. This isn't a life-threatening situation, so we should use our interpersonal and social skills to deal with the conflict and remain feeling calm. It is natural that you will initially feel highly aroused by this kind of situation, but an effective system, with a healthy vagus brake, will quickly turn this arousal off, and the brain calibrates that it is just your neighbour kicking off again, and nothing life threatening. Very quickly, you *should* revert to using your calm, social defence to deal with him, and anyone else. You should use your social defence skills to assert yourself, calmly and easily, listen and respond, using an appropriate tone of voice and facial expression to let that person know you are not intimidated, that you are not affected by their rage, and you can then calmly negotiate a solution. The other person gets the measure of you, calms down, or stomps off. There is no need to activate the red track, your sympathetic system, the chimp, when it detects you are safe. Hence, our nonverbal signals are *critical* in maintaining health and enabling your body to stay in the green track, physically unaffected by activity or discord.

Porges argues that because we evolved to be social creatures, we physically *need* other people to be nurturing as it activates our own healthy vagal system (the green track). We are physically soothed and nurtured by other peoples' friendly facial expressions, intonation of voice, and gestures. "The neural circuit for social interaction and social engagement is the same neural circuit that supports health, growth and restoration." (Porges, 2014 p.12). This is why it is so important to have people around you who are encouraging, positive and supportive of you, not only during recovery, but always. You do not want to be surrounded by sceptic tones, hostility, and disapproving faces during recovery and thereafter. Likewise, during recovery, you don't need marshmallowing tones from others, as that implies you are fragile and incapable. If we detect an unfriendly tone of voice or facial expression, we then need to activate our *own* defence skills using our facial expression, tone of voice, posture, and gestures to deal with it, which ensures we stay in the healthy, calm thrive mode.

Porges also showed that some people *lack* the necessary Social Skills for Defence and therefore turn on the powerful defence mechanisms for Fight, Flight, and Freeze automatically and inappropriately. Have you ever noticed that throughout your life, you don't always stay in the healthy, calm mode when dealing with certain people or situations? When level 1 doesn't resolve the problem, or you don't have the nonverbal social skills repertoire, the body turns on level 2, the high arousal chimp mode. The neurological dysfunction probably didn't start with getting a virus; for most people the wrong systems had been activated for years. Without our first defence strategies, we only had the chimp and reptile to rely on.

LEVEL 2: The Mammalian Response. Also known as The Chimp, or the red branch on the diagram; our Sympathetic Nervous System. We have been discussing throughout the book how this system is malfunctioning in CFS. When it fires off, we are thrown into high arousal to mobilise, to get away or to fight the demon. If you were a car, you would be hitting the high revs, and going into the red zone. It is appropriate occasionally to accelerate out of danger, but it is dangerous to stay in those revs too long because you will burn out the engine. Imagine if we had to turn on that system every time we are exposed to conflict, fell out with someone, and had to deal with unreasonable demands or discord? No wonder the body burns out. Our physiology is over-reacting in non-life-threatening events far too often, and therefore putting it out of balance. Sadly, when we live in this arousal mode for too long, the human social mode is so deactivated that it starts to misinterpret other peoples' facial expressions and tone of voice as unfriendly threats. Maybe that is why some people trapped in this physiology during illness become defensive and think people are blaming them for being ill? Clearly, when we are ill, fight and flight doesn't resolve our symptoms, so level 3 takes over.

LEVEL 3: The Reptilian Response. Also referred to as the grey branch in the diagram above or our Dorsal Vagus. The ultimate defence mechanism kicks in to immobilise us and shut us down. Furthermore, Porges explains in his NICABM seminar that:

> *"after a single traumatic incident, the person can be normal before the traumatic event but then, as the body shuts down, they start having symptoms of lower gut issues, can't deal with proximity of people, become hypersensitive to low frequency sounds and even has severe issues of fibromyalgia and blood pressure regulation.... neural regulation is different afterwards".* (2015 p.15)

The initial crash and disability with CFS and Long Covid are hugely traumatic, and this will contribute to neural irregulation and sustained reptilian activity, post-trauma. In this mode, the body will tick over and remain safe but be immobile. This is the experience of having CFS; our bodies are running at a sustainable level to keep us alive but nothing more. To use our car analogy, imagine if your body were a car; your engine is ticking over, but you are stationary. You can't move, but *there is no damage*. When we lack the healthy first line of defence in our repertoire, the defensive social skills, then we can only "up the ante" and rely on the chimp or reptile defences to get us into fight and flight or freeze. As Porges explains this in his book, *The Polyvagal Theory* (2011 p.265), "under most challenges in our environment, we initially react with our newest system..if the circuit does not satisfy our biobehavioral quest for safety, an older circuit spontaneously reacts..as our last option we reflexively trigger the oldest circuit.".

Most of the clients I have worked with display *very competent* social skills in terms of interacting with others. They are adept at being warm, friendly and using the right tone of voice to engage with people. In fact, they are so skilled at engaging, caring, empathy and attachment that they make excellent teachers, nurses, midwives, social workers and doctors. Indeed, many people with CFS are professionals in these areas. It is only their *defence* social engagement skills that are missing, the ones Porges calls our human social engagement defence. I would suggest that most people with CFS have not used their defence social skills enough because:

- We weren't taught to use them.
- We were repressed from using them.
- They weren't effective when dealing with threatening people who held power over us. Trying to negotiate with dominant, unreasonable people doesn't work.
- Long term, repetitive conflict and disharmony means the other defences must kick in, as the solution isn't solved by talking or being assertive.

However, we can learn the skills now and use them to stay in the healthy green track.

Learning Social Defence Skills

Defence skills are our first line of defence to protect us from overload and being physically affected by others. They should be automatic and easy, just like smiling or having good manners. To stay robust and healthy you need to:

- Focus on your own health throughout life.
- Know your limitations - all humans have a tolerance level.
- Know what is reasonable to stay healthy.
- Have a deep sense of self-worth, knowing how you deserve to be treated.
- Be self-assured and keep clarity.
- Be unaffected by other peoples' bad behaviour by staying in level one, on the green track.
- Use your nonverbal signals to defend yourself and stay strong.
- Express yourself in a challenging situation and be able to answer back.

- Speak up because your opinion and health matters as much as anyone else's.
- Be non-compliant in situations when it would be unhealthy to comply.
- Set boundaries and say no to unreasonable demands.
- Refuse to take on further load when you are already functioning near full capacity.

All these needs involve level one social defence skills. If you didn't learn these defence skills because they weren't part of your family or cultural norms, or because you weren't allowed to be assertive, then you will lack the primary armour for dealing robustly with life. Human mode defences are our outer protective shell, our thick skin. Without which we are physiologically affected by people and situations, especially if we are naturally gentle, caring and have deep empathy for others. Many people who lack this coat of armour have great lives, because they live only in nurturing environments, so don't need them. However, others are exposed to regular overload, abusive, controlling situations or life events, where we do need social defence skills to deal with it.

Lacking the ability to set limits, stand your ground, deal with confrontation, and negotiate terms, means people activate high arousal or take on too much. This, combined with a propensity to have an easily aroused adaptive system and exposure to long term unfavourable conditions, can lead to exhaustion, fatigue and CFS, as well as other illnesses.

Here are some common conditioned responses which, of course, are *not* exclusive to people having CFS or Long Covid. Every human being has conditioned responses because 80% of life is conditioning. Once established, triggers activate your response, and you have no control over it, until you develop an awareness and commit to stopping habits consciously, as you will learn to do shortly. You may want to consider which situations you struggle to use your social defences and resort to animal survival modes. Triggers are very powerful, as we learnt from Pavlov. I could run a behaviour centre with the persistent threat of aggression or hostility and be okay, and yet I couldn't deal with constant discord in social and personal situations. We learn professional skills as adults; the youngsters were my trigger for being professional. In the home environment we are conditioned to respond in the ways we learnt early on. As a lovely and brilliantly successful consultant with Long Covid said, "you don't expect loved ones to turn on you". Think carefully about your triggers so you are better prepared and can make conscious choices in future.

Common Patterns

Being Physically Affected by Others: Every person I have ever worked with has said that the one thing they would like to change is to stop being physically affected by other people's behaviour. Clearly if you didn't learn defence skills or weren't able to use them during early years development, you are left with only the chimp and reptile responses; physically aroused or immobilised by triggers.

Have a think about what triggers you to feel physically affected by another person's actions. Is it the facial expression, tone of voice, or gestures? You will use your Traffic Lights procedure to stop automatic responses and be able to deal with anything. It is important to learn your own limitations, delegate and set boundaries to stay healthy. This is especially true if you are a carer dealing with loved ones and leaving isn't an option.

The Enthusiast: Enthusiasts have a great zest for life and feel invincible. They like being busy and stimulated by work, hobbies, studying or socialising and often don't know the art of relaxing. They say yes to everything, lacking a clear perspective of what is reasonable. They will be frustrated if an injury or illness sets them back and slows them down, which often causes them to get going too quickly whilst the body is still recovering. They often run the "boom and bust" pattern during recovery.

It is great to be an enthusiast when fully healthy, but the problem is when it goes too far; when you can't stop, even when the load has become unrealistic. Do you lack an awareness of time and motion, thinking you can just squeeze another thing in or stretch out time? Seriously review your response to load. Check with others if you are doing more than is reasonable and sustainable. You can do things for years, but after decades, it may affect the body.

EXERCISE: Keep a note on how long you think tasks will take, and then record how long they actually take. It will help you develop a reality check and better time management.

A large part of social defence skills is being able to set boundaries if you reasonably can't do something. What would happen if you did set a reasonable boundary for demands, even if it means letting people down?

Firefighters - The Rescuer: These are caring, empathetic people who are forever going to someone's rescue or who wants help. They stay loyal to people who need rescuing, often offering financial help or doing jobs, when they don't have extra supplies to give. The problem comes when you can't say no, and you feel compelled to help. Are you capable of saying no? How would you feel if you said no? Bad, guilty, anxious, selfish? Again, unhealthy beliefs ("I have to help") and inappropriate emotions can get us stuck in unhealthy patterns. Is there really no one else, or can the person work it out on their own when you don't jump to the rescue? It is empowering for other people when they realise that they are capable and able to resolve the crisis themselves. Do you trust that they are competent, that they will get through this or learn from it? Without boundaries and defence skills, the firefighter can easily become physically, mentally, emotionally, and socially drained. The Traffic Lights procedure at the end of the chapter will enable you to use healthier responses to situations.

Accommodating Unreasonable Behaviour: Accommodating loved ones is normal and healthy when it is reciprocal and loving. However, continually accommodating others to avoid disharmony isn't healthy. Compliant people lack the defence skill to be non-compliant, and challenge when necessary. Again, these patterns have been shaped by experiences, such as living with a powerhouse who wouldn't be challenged, or it comes from low self-esteem. It is normal for children to be compliant and to fit in with adults, but if you only learnt to be compliant, you will lack the defence skills needed for adulting.

Humans are always trying to stay in the calm, parasympathetic nervous system; we do *whatever it takes* to avoid confrontation and upset. When you learn assertiveness and robust social skills however, you can live healthily and stay calm, without using accommodating strategies.

Can't Hurt Other People's Feelings (even if they are behaving badly): How many of us believe it is wrong to hurt the other person? We feel shame, guilt and discomfort if we do. How many of us struggle to tell other people that they are wrong, being unreasonable or unfair? What would it take for you to set boundaries, to say "enough"? When you are kind, it may seem abhorrent to hurt someone else's feelings, even though that person is hurting you, overloading you or taking you for granted. You may think it is appropriate to challenge a child but wrong to challenge an adult. When you don't have all the social skills an unhealthy balance develops. Our social tool kit must have all the tools needed to be a robust and healthy adult; you can be a nice person and still be assertive. Counsellors teach that "anger is your dignity", and that it is okay to be angry sometimes when someone is doing something to you that isn't good for you. Every human is born with the capacity to be angry, but anger can be suppressed, either by others, or because you learnt early on that anger is bad and vowed never to show it. Dignified anger to protect yourself is appropriate when you are being hurt, taken for granted, or being treated badly.

Empathy is an essential part of socialisation; without empathy, we would be narcissistic sociopaths. However, empathy can become a problem, rather than a useful tool, when you care more for them than your own health and wellbeing. Were you taught as a child to make excuses for bad behaviour and in so doing, became brilliant at putting up with bad behaviour? For some, living with bad behaviour was the norm, and your role in life was to be the peacekeeper or accommodator.

Did you spread yourself too thin looking after others? Often other people are simply unaware how much they put on others, oblivious to their own pattern, so it is up to you to set the boundaries. Begin by establishing this healthy belief, "I can be a nice person and still set healthy boundaries- I matter as much as anyone else".

Highly Conscientious: Every Persian rug is made with a faulty stitch as a way to remind Muslims that only God is perfect. As humans we shouldn't try to be God or get everything right. To err is human. It is okay to say and do the wrong thing, then aspire to improve.

Overly conscientious people work hard and try harder and harder to do their best in everything they do, whether it is parenting, work or home- then become overloaded as a result. If you are given a target or job, do you automatically assume you should be able to do it? If you are told to do something, do you think that means you *have* to do it, no matter how unreasonable it actually is? Many people have become overloaded because they were overly conscientious, overly compliant, always optimising. They believe that it is right to be conscientious, to optimise and achieve, whatever they are given. Do you assume, because someone said to do it, you should do it? Do you accept their judgement rather than trust your own judgement? Could you imagine yourself saying, "No, I can't"?

When we are programmed to be compliant, lack self-consideration and the social defence skills to challenge other people, it is easy to get overloaded. My bosses asked me to take on a full-time position, on top of my already demanding full-time job, because they were desperate. I agreed, because legally we had to meet certain requirements and there was "no-one else" who could take it on, apparently. What should have been a one term cover turned into 18 months and doing two full-time jobs was exhausting, on top of running a home, a family, and a difficult situation. When I crashed, my boss said, "You should never have taken on that other job". When I said, "You were the ones who begged me to do it", she replied, "Yes, but we weren't thinking straight". Bosses are human and make mistakes like the rest of us, so it is essential to stop the automatic pattern of feeling you should, even if authority or loved ones demand it, because it can cause unreasonable load. When you don't have the human social defence skills to challenge others, you activate the chimp and the reptile over and over again because they are your only defence mechanisms. If you can't reason with your boss or other significant person, consider alternative options. It seems that many "optimisers" think they are judged as not being professional if they say no. Organisations can easily play on the conscientiousness of staff- one only needs to look at recent events in the NHS to see it was dependent on the good-will of conscientious staff. But at what cost to staff, who may vote with their feet to survive.

Beliefs and values are the drivers. Conscientious people care too much. Start with reviewing your standards, your expectations, and beliefs. Watch out for also setting unrealistic targets for yourself. 70% success in everything you do is plenty. Become more aware of the triggers that fire off the pattern and then commit to learning a different response and take control.

Successful people know their limitations and say no. Get rid of the belief, "I should be able to do this if it has been given to me" and start thinking rationally. Consider, is it realistic? Do you have the skill set to express yourself and set boundaries? Truly healthy people care less. That doesn't mean they don't care about things; they may care deeply but they also care less about failing or upsetting people. Self-esteem isn't hard wired to success. They have the skills to say no, to refuse or to challenge, thereby managing their load and keeping it healthy. They focus less on others and have the calm robustness to challenge. They don't care if someone doesn't like what they say or do, as long as they feel comfortable with it; so, they have no emotional, intellectual, or social load. Often, they delegate or refuse to do certain chores at home, or in work, thus taking the load off themselves. They don't have a higher threshold than other people, they just make sure they don't function to full capacity and go beyond their tolerance level. They have self-esteem, self-worth and have the defence skills to stay in the healthy track. Crucially, when they live in the calm vagal system, they can think straight and assess the situation accurately. In my experience, people respect you more if you stand up to them, especially bullies.

Repress how we are: In his book, *Why Zebras Don't Get Ulcers* (2004), Sapolsky shows how the repressed personality is affected by fatigue. These are people appearing fine on the surface, the brave soldier who carries on regardless, doing a sterling job in everything they do without complaint or expression, smiling even if they are struggling. It is the Graceful Swan, calm but paddling like fury on the inside, gradually going under. Someone or something in the environment taught them to repress any negative emotion or weakness, never to complain, and to only talk of positive things. They were taught to put on a brave face and that expressing any negative emotion or weakness is unacceptable. It was imperative not to make a fuss or show struggles to the outside world. Society still keeps men in the "man box", stiff upper lip, and tragically, so many men who repress how they really feel but don't talk about it then commit suicide, when life gets too much.

Keeping going in adversity isn't a bad thing; it builds resilience and strength. There is no such thing as a good or bad strategy. What matters is balance and being adaptable. It is good to keep going, to be resilient, but it is not good if you are going under and don't have the tools to express yourself, get support and effect change. So many millennials, so many men caught in the "man box", and so many women, are trying to keep going under duress, not realising that the PIES they are juggling are actually ten times greater than other people's load. So many people are also struggling but say nothing, until they get ill. Other people may be doing the same job but going back home with no responsibilities or strife, and so have time to relax, to sleep, to wind down and counteract the load at work. You may be going back to a very different scenario. Furthermore, if you have no secure support network to confide in, as is the case for many men, or if you have been isolated from friends by a partner, you will go under on your own. The social and emotional support from friends and family would have acted as a buffer. Many adults try to keep going as normal because they want to be strong and be good role models for their children. As we know, when supplies run dry, this can lead to fatigue, CFS or other illnesses.

People who do life the right way express themselves and put their hands up to say, "I am struggling", or "I can't do this", "I need help". They delegate to others and ask for help. They do not perceive this as a weakness and don't go beyond their threshold tolerance level. The ability to speak up and express yourself is an essential defence skill, combating overload.

When a repressed person crashes with CFS or can't recover from viruses, it is devastating because they value strength, the ability to keep going, and unconsciously feel that weakness is something to be ashamed of. It also explains why so many people with CFS want it to be caused by a virus; having a virus does not imply weakness. For me, being publicly exposed as weak was excruciating, nearly as bad as the crash itself. The jibes that I was "putting it on" to get sympathy made it even worse. When our identity is to be calm and carry on, when we don't want a fuss, don't want to worry others, hate drama and don't want to be seen as a victim, it is soul destroying to crash so dramatically, so publicly, and get attention for all the wrong reasons. But it was also a lesson that I had to learn; I have nothing to be ashamed of. If another person had carried my load, they would have collapsed years before I did.

I doubt someone having a heart condition or a stroke feels shame or is made to feel they are weak and yet they are influenced by the autonomic system, like CFS. A human being should never be raised to be ashamed of themselves; they need to be proud of themselves and have unconditional self-worth, crucial building blocks for defence against life's challenges. Whoever instilled shame in children was misguided, wrong, not the children. Thankfully today there is a much greater emphasis on teaching children that their actions may not have been appropriate but they, as people, are worthy. I hope by exposing my struggle with the shame of crashing and deciding I have nothing to be ashamed of, it enables you to release yourself and do what it takes to break free and be robust forever. Be glad you can rectify the malfunctioning autonomic system that was activated over and over again through circumstances and perpetuated by the illness. Be proud that you can effect changes, develop the first line of defence armoury, and don't wait for a pill to recover.

There will be an exercise later in the chapter and in the online videos at www.resettothrive.co.uk to help you stop the shame and access self-worth. For further reading, an excellent book worth checking out is *Destructive Emotions and how to overcome them. A dialogue with the Dalai Lama* (2015) by Daniel Goleman. Also look at *I Heart Me* (2015) by David Hamilton to understand why negative emotions and repression are damaging, and why we need to express ourselves authentically to physically heal.

Clearly, all these patterns lead to increased load, physically, mentally, emotionally, and socially, taking you beyond the healthy threshold. Without the first level of defence skills to set boundaries, we say yes to demands and tasks, have unhealthy boundaries, cannot challenge others, or assert our needs and rely on the chimp or reptile as our only defence systems. Inappropriate caring, accommodating, conscientiousness, being affected by others, and a wobbly self-assuredness can all increase the load we take on. Being prickly and defensive at any sniff of criticism or disapproval will increase our social, mental, and emotional load.

We need robust defence skills to act as a buffer, deflect the onslaught and manage overload. To stay healthy, we have to skill up, show up, become assertive, express ourselves, set healthy boundaries, have an unconditional regard for ourselves and have clarity. We need to see when others are running unhealthy patterns and protect ourselves, always ensuring we stay in the calm, healthy, parasympathetic system. We have to learn to be at ease in any situation, knowing we are safe and okay.

It is very likely that your environmental conditions were persistent and chronic. It is not possible to thrive in situations that are unhealthy, so even when you learn the defence skills, if you cannot change the situation, it is better to leave and find healthier relationships, employers and environmental conditions.

How Social Defence Skills Develop

Porges talked about the first line of defence as being social; defence skills for conflict resolution, including assertiveness, expression, self-assuredness and robustness, and an ability to say no and set boundaries.

It is normal for a toddler to display instinctive responses before they develop the human social defence skills. So how do we learn those skills? Just as we learn all the other social skills. When these social defence skills are learnt early on, especially within five to seven years of age, a child doesn't have to rely only on the fight, flight, or freeze instincts they are born with. When we are surrounded with a friendly pack, we are protected, and within our tribe we are taught how to develop and use the skills to defend ourselves in the outside world. Children who were not brought up to be scared, put down or controlled, but instead raised in a safe and loving atmosphere, are blessed. They are allowed to have their voices heard and valued, to have an opinion, to express themselves, openly and easily, feeling loved and equal. They learnt not only to be assertive, but that assertiveness is normal, essential, healthy, and safe. They were reasoned with. They learnt that what they think matters, that it is safe to argue your case and sometimes win, that they matter, and they can recognise when other people are wrong or behaving wrongly. They learnt critical social and emotional literacy that will serve them throughout life. When a child develops deep foundations of self-worth and self-assured, they value themselves, have dignity and self-respect and therefore are much more likely to be able to set boundaries, knowing how they expect to be treated; they know what is acceptable and what isn't and they are self-assured enough to express it, standing firm against others, using their highly-tuned defence skills. Just to reiterate, consider if:

- You missed out on this stage of development because these skills weren't familiar in your environment and the other family members lacked them too.

- You were prevented from developing these defence skills because standing up for yourself and defending yourself was forbidden in your environment.
- You were exposed to tones of voice, expressions and gestures that scared or unnerved you in the early years, when you only had the chimp and reptile instincts to rely on. This became the default mode.
- You have a propensity to be hijacked by the arousal system or freeze mode, and the vagal brake didn't kick in quickly enough, so you couldn't respond as you would have liked to at the time.
- You had level 1 defence skills and used them in normal situations, but they were no match for the conditions you were living in or working under. You cannot reason with people who are running dysfunctional patterns or set reasonable boundaries. Therefore, base defences were activated again and again.

It is not your fault if you didn't develop certain social skills. Without an effective first line of defence, you go into the world with only the inappropriate chimp and reptile to assist you. It is like taking a sledgehammer to crack a nut and the body is not meant to keep going in over arousal or shock. Turning on level two and level three defences is fine for fighting tigers but not fine if the trigger is a constant part of your life, whether at work or home.

Many people do learn to be assertive and self-assured when they go into training or the workplace, which stands them in good stead for work triggers and social settings. They are competent at work but struggle with relationships because of early conditioning or life experiences. This is the stimulus response we discussed, salivating to the bell or reacting to a tone of voice.

Becoming More Resourceful

We are going to stop being triggered by other people's facial expression, tone of voice or gestures and instead stay clear headed. We will use our tone of voice, facial expressions, gestures and posture to demonstrate to others that we have dignity, we know what is acceptable and what isn't.

That we know how we deserve to be treated, can express how things need to be, can set boundaries, and not put up with bad behaviour from others.

Before we move onto breaking habits of a lifetime, or patterns that have become automatic, just consider:

- What would happen if you did say no to someone and refused to do what they asked?
- Always think; what would happen if I did? What would happen if I didn't?

In a relationship, would the person walk away? Would they retaliate even more? At work, do you imagine you would be sacked? Would you be making it harder for others?

Reasonable people will realise they have made unrealistic requests when you challenge them and be fine about it. If not, you seriously need to consider if they are good for sustainable health and if this is a viable environment. Living in fear of being sacked, being disliked, being rejected or abandoned will only feed the chimp and is untenable. Know what is healthy, what is right for you. We need to take responsibility for our own well-being.

Beliefs and values that we take for granted and think are beneficial, can sometimes get us in trouble if we hold onto them when it isn't appropriate. Chapter 1 highlighted how beliefs drive our actions, and they make us behave in certain ways. Become mindful of any beliefs and values that may be affecting your well-being and how you do life. There is no such thing as a good or bad belief, just whether it is appropriate in any given situation. You may believe it is good to help, but not if that person wants your blood. Our values underpin how we live life and are very powerful, so consider being more adaptable. Loyalty is good, but not to someone who isn't healthy for you. Being a Good Samaritan is lovely, but not when you feed an incorrigible taker, or wear yourself into the ground.

Just as importantly, your perception of events needs to be healthy. This is why in recovery you needed to perceive activity and symptoms as being okay, so the amygdala relearnt that everything is safe and didn't need to turn on survival mode. Just because it *feels* scary, doesn't mean it actually *is* scary. As you become mindful of this, you will recalibrate things that had been perceived as a threat, to now being of little consequence. Whatever you notice yourself doing that isn't healthy, you are going to stop and practise healthy responses.

Using the Traffic Lights System to Break Patterns and Improve Skills

Even in the most nurturing environment, there will be times when other people are not thinking straight, when they are overloaded and just want to offload on someone else. There will be times when you need to deal with discord, disagreement, bullies, or dysfunctional behaviour in others. Hence, you are going to improve your social defence skills and set boundaries, so that you are not overloaded with PIES. We need a wide range of resources to adapt to any situation, "a blade of grass in a gale and a gale against a strong wall". It is not sufficient to only have caring and engaging social skills.

Awareness: As you know, the first stage in changing responses is to be aware of triggers, and moving patterns from unconscious, automatic states to conscious, deliberate states. We know the power of triggers; they turn on our physiology and make us feel certain ways, automatically and unconsciously, just like dogs salivating to a ringing bell. Throughout the book you have been practising mindfulness, approaching everything as a detached, intrigued observer. As you become more aware of the triggers and unhealthy responses, jot down the patterns you want to stop.

Simply become mindful. Start to notice other people's facial expressions and tone of voice as a distant observer. See things differently: If they are angry, see them going red like a raging bull, booming like an empty vessel, ranting like a toddler. Just notice how ridiculous it looks. As you practise mindfulness, you will notice that other people's patterns are often nothing to do with you. You can rise above it, see it for what it is; it is just stuff. They cannot harm you when you are dissociated from them and then it will give you the space to respond how you want to. Let them take responsibility for their own patterns, it is not your job. If they want to change, they will seek out all the information and help they can to change.

Red, Amber, Green: First, we will review the whole procedure and then we will use it for specific examples; you can then apply it to any inappropriate responses. When I did Traffic Lights with young people, they found it easier to put three coloured spots on the floor to remind them which stage they were at in the procedure.

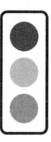

STOP

THINK. ENGAGE HIGHER BRAIN AND CHOOSE HOW TO RESPOND

PROCEED ONCE YOU HAVE ACCESSED APPROPRIATE RESPONSES

RED = STOP. Recognise the response you want to stop. Use the tone of voice, facial expression, posture, and gestures already discussed to do a definite, firm stop. Feel what it feels like to say stop. Some people use other words, so find something that resonates with you. Ensure that everything about your movements, tone and expression is deliberate and controlled. The tone needs to match what you want: energised for energy, slow and calm for calmness.

AMBER = THINK AND ENGAGE YOUR CONSCIOUS BRAIN. As the higher brain engages, you are going to talk to yourself in a kind way, really meaning what you are saying. Get into a habit of saying the same thing each time, so it becomes a habit, quick and easy.

The job of the thinking brain is to be rational, to assess the situation, make a judgement and solve a problem. The following example is a typical process people say on amber to activate the thinking brain and allow it to override the lower, instinctive protective brain.

"Is it useful to be like this?
Absolutely not. I don't need it and I will decide how I want to be.
I want to be healthy, robust, and strong.
You can do this. Focus.
How do I need to be right now?
I need to fire off Healthy States".
Come on. You *can* do this.

Throughout the book, you have already affected change. Therefore, if you think you can't do this exercise to switch states, recognise it is just the chimp chattering. Young children do this and find it fun. Focus on what you are doing and what you want, not on what you don't want. Notice that on amber, you are consciously assessing the situation, you are encouraging yourself, building your confidence, making conscious decisions, and getting on with the job. This is about being calm and determined; no shouting, no panic, just switching from one track to another and consciously living.

GREEN = PROCEED AND ASSOCIATE INTO A HEALTHY STATE.
Before you step into the healthy state, it would be useful to compose yourself, to take a breath and use your focus gesture, either the blinkered horse or the single hand going straight as an arrow from the nose forward. Say "Focus". This is for you to focus on the exercise. Nothing else exists for the few moments you are doing this exercise. When you become brilliant at performing this technique from NLP, it only takes a couple of minutes and you can learn to do it anytime you need it, especially when you learn to do it subtly. Elite sports people can stand at the starting line or in the dressing room before performing and get themselves into the best state for what they are about to do. It just takes practise. If you are not getting results, stop and revise. Look at www.resettothrive.co.uk for demonstrations. Do not practise doing it the wrong way because that will only reinforce the unhealthy state and make you give up. Record the instructions on your phone, so you can listen as you practise.

- Close your eyes and take yourself back to anytime when you responded the way you want to respond now. You are just going to make the brain remember it so it can fire off the healthy pathways again.

- Step into that moment again, and access the *exact* tone of voice, facial expression, gestures and the position of your head in that moment. If you are walking, stand still but feel the pace and the pressure on your feet. If you are sitting in the memory, feel yourself sitting, in the exact posture, or actually sit down.

- In the present moment, notice what you are wearing, seeing, hearing, touching, smelling, tasting. Fire off the sensory input associated with this wonderful moment. Feel what it feels like in this moment, and fire off that feeling and notice where you feel it. Let it spread to every part of you.

- As soon as you access the healthy state, add a symbol to associate with this peak moment (this is called an anchor, or a conditioned stimulus, essentially just something you learn to respond to). It could be a colour, a shape, a sound, a piece of music or song, or click your fingers or squeeze your fist. Like the bell to food, as you repeat this, you will be able to trigger physiology with this association and feel the healthy state.

- Take your mind off this moment; think about cabbages! Then as you bring back this symbol, notice how quickly you access the healthy state.

- As you open your eyes, notice that you have won the Battle of the Brains. You have overcome the chimp, the reptile and fired off the healthy human pathways again. Use the social defence skills from now on to break habits.

Alternative Responses to the Automatic Habits

Here is a list of some of the patterns you may want to change but there may be others, specific to your circumstances.

I want to stop unhealthy states	I need to access healthy states
Body shutting down	Get the body working, energy and strength
Body in arousal, wired, nausea, pain, tension	Get the body in a calm, healthy mode
Not sure of myself, don't know my own mind	Be self-assured; to know what is right for me
Fearful	Need to trust I am okay, I am competent
Anxious	Anticipate I can do. Belief and trust. Be excited
Accommodate others too much	Focus on own needs and set boundaries
Affected by others, feeling like a child, fearful or inferior	Be unaffected by others. Adult to adult. Use defence skills appropriate for the situation. Stop caring what people think- you know who you are and they can have their own opinion, Let go of hurt, within minutes of being triggered
Not good enough. Berate myself- unfriendly to myself.	Unconditionally good enough. Be your own best friend, with friendly nonverbal signals.
Lack deep inner, calm confidence. Believe others	Confidence
Care too much	Care less; don't care, nothing matters that much
Overwhelmed	Clear Headed, prioritise, get a realistic perspective
Can't speak up and say what I need to say	Have a voice; express yourself. Be confidently assertive

Guilt and shame	Pride/ dignity, self-worth, relaxed body. When you know you have done nothing to intentionally harm others
Worry about people I love	Trust they are resourceful; believe in them. Support
Can't say no, even when I want to	Find a time you can say no easily
Enthusiastic then exhausted	Stop, slow down, think, is this reasonable? Step into clear headed, logical, realistic balance
Firefighter, the rescuer	Setting boundaries, knowing limitations. Trust that others are competent and capable and don't always need rescuing. Access other support for them.
Personalise everything	It's not my problem. They have issues, it's not about me.
Can't answer back when challenged or when people are angry	Have clarity about the situation. Dignified anger. Express yourself easily, be assertive, have your perspective on the situation. Tell people if they are behaving inappropriately and set boundaries. Care less about their bad behaviour - not your problem. Give them a wide berth.

Applying the Traffic Lights Procedure: Examples for you to Follow

Example 1. Setting Boundaries:

Firstly, notice what the triggers are. Is it a word someone says? Or is it a tone or an expression that makes you accommodate, even when you are already overloaded? It is kind and considerate to help each other but not if you are already overloaded or they are in the habit of using people. It took me years to work out why I felt compelled to say yes when people said, "can you?" To me, saying no was unkind, selfish, and made me feel guilty. The reason it takes so long to work out our response to triggers is because our beliefs and values are completely unconscious. Whatever we learnt years ago, has just become an automatic response, not a conscious decision.

It is really worth making your beliefs and values conscious now; sometimes they need tweaking. Whilst I still really value helping others and value kindness, it is not selfish or bad to consider yourself in the equation. I will, if I can, but not if I get overloaded in the process. People are often not being inconsiderate or unkind when they ask favours or make demands; sometimes they just need to get something done quickly and are not thinking about the impact on asking others. Sometimes they are anxious or lack confidence and that makes them needy. It doesn't matter what their intention is, what matters is how you choose to respond.

It is the unconscious beliefs and values that drive your responses to triggers, so do become more aware of them and decide consciously to change your automatic reaction to a trigger. We started our journey by considering our beliefs about CFS and recovery because they are powerful drivers in everything we do.

Get into the habit of noticing the phrases or the tone that triggers you. This will give you time to become conscious, instead of just reacting. In the beginning you may not be able to stop the autopilot response, but you are becoming aware, which is the first step in change. Initially, when you are thrown into an old pattern, it is best to take yourself off for a few minutes so that you can do the Traffic Lights procedure, whether it's in a loo, or a quiet room. If you are on the phone, say you will call them back. Anything to gain time, to take yourself off and do a manual reset.

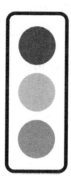

STOP unconscious habits

THINK. Engage higher, conscious brain

PROCEED. Step into how you want to be and <u>then</u> carry on

RED = STOP. Press the Pause Button. Give your brain time to engage. Use your nonverbal signals and be completely committed and already feel you are taking control.

AMBER = THINK. Engage your brain. Decide if it is useful running the same old pattern or would it be more useful to choose how you want to respond. Remind yourself you can do this; you did it before and you can step into a healthier state again. I say to myself:

> "Is it useful being like this? Absolutely not. How would I rather be? I would rather be able to say no and set healthy boundaries. Come on, you can do that by stepping into anytime when you have boundaries and can say no. Focus only on that moment."

GREEN = ACTION. Take yourself back to a time when it is easy to say no. Always choose something easy or memorable. Bring up a time when someone asked if you want a cup of tea, and you could say no. Or a time when someone asked you to go for a drink and you declined. Essentially, anytime when you were relaxed about saying no. Now, step into that person, and have your expression, gestures, posture, tone of voice and actions exactly as they are in this moment when you are saying no. Take in what you are wearing, seeing, hearing, touching, doing, smelling, tasting, whatever is relevant and feel what it feels like saying no, completely at ease and relaxed.

Pair the healthy state with a symbol; it could be a visual object, a colour, a sound, a song or piece of music or something kinaesthetic like a tap, a click, or a clap. Think of cabbages, then bring back the symbol and notice how quickly the healthy states return. Once you have refreshed that feeling and fired it off again, you can then, and only then, return to the current scenario, as a person with healthy social defence skills, and just say no.

Example 2. Stop Being Physically Affected by Others and Express Yourself Easily:

This is a real scenario from one of my clients:

> "I had only been with my new partner for a few months when, in a coffee shop, he snapped at me for taking too long deciding which coffee I wanted. Being snapped at by someone who, two seconds before had been so sweet, was a shock. I felt physically upset and did my usual pattern, said nothing and conformed; I ordered the first coffee I saw on the list, to stop him being annoyed. My colleagues wouldn't have believed my response, because they see me as this competent, capable woman, who I am most of the time. Anger and getting told off, puts me straight back in my box. I had done Jan's course on breaking patterns, so I excused myself, went off to the loo and took a deep breath to calm down. Then, I looked in the mirror. I spoke to myself kindly (and very quietly), just as I would when talking to a friend:
>
> Stop. That's enough; you are not a child anymore; you can do this.
>
> Think. What if he were in the wrong, and you had done nothing wrong? How do you want to be? I want to go back

and talk to him like an adult, it's as easy as saying, "Do you want a cup of tea" to your friend. You behave like an adult all the time when you are not being told off. You can do this. Be how you want to be. I want to be at ease and have a voice. Close your eyes and step into being yourself, with your friend, Anna.

Proceed. Take yourself back to a time when you are an adult, with other adults and have a voice, that moment with Anna, when you can talk freely.

Once I felt back to normal, I decided if he doesn't like me having an opinion and saying how I saw the situation then, tough, I don't need someone like that in my life.

I went back to the table, took a breath, and recited, 'Do you want a cup of tea?', silently in my head. Then, I said what I needed to say, calmly and clearly. 'When you snapped at me about the coffee, I was really shocked. I didn't expect you to get so angry over nothing and I don't need that. I wait for you to choose different beers, so you can wait for me to choose different coffees.'

His response was extraordinary. He said, 'I'm so glad you spoke to me about it, instead of building it up into a big deal and I'm sorry I snapped, I just don't get this fuss about coffee. You're completely right; I hadn't thought of it that way before.' I had never been with a reasonable partner before, so this response was amazing. Since then, he doesn't get annoyed about all the different coffees on offer!

I learnt then that I always need to communicate effectively in challenging situations and put a conscious stop on unhealthy autopilot patterns that I have carried with me since I was little. I also learnt that life is easier when I focus on my needs and wants and not on keeping them calm or doing as I'm told because they say so. And thankfully, I discovered that he is a lovely, reasonable man who sometimes gets it wrong, like the

rest of us. We can work things out when we are reasonable
grown-ups, just by communicating honestly and effectively."

Instead of dancing to his tune, she decided to dance to her own tune and not jump to his commands. This lady not only changed her habitual response to being snapped at, but she learnt to value her own opinion, to trust herself and to recognise that *just because people say things, doesn't mean it is true.* They are just opinions and beliefs - he believed that nobody should make such a big deal about coffee just because he didn't like coffee. She stopped thinking she was doing something wrong, or it was her fault, when others were angry at her, and realised others are wrong too sometimes.

She learnt to focus on herself, her needs, and her well-being. Change isn't about changing other people. She learnt to say how she deserved to be treated and wasn't going to put up with anything less. Accessing defence skills enabled her to set very clear boundaries about how things need to be, for her to stay in the relationship, happy and healthy. She wasn't prepared to live in an unhealthy environment and decided that she would only be with reasonable, stable, and secure people in future, who enabled her to thrive, feel at ease and live in the healthy autonomic system. Being around friendly people really is important for staying healthy.

It is fascinating that she always had the skills in her repertoire, they just weren't turned on by this particular trigger (the angry voice telling her she is in trouble). All she had to do was transfer skills from when she uses them naturally, asking if anyone wants a cup of tea, to a situation where the *trigger* had made her back down, putting her back in her box, doing as she was told. Break free from any box you were put in.

Everyone has all the resources; it is just we couldn't use them when the trigger threw us into bad states. How often have you been thrown into bad states and wished you had responded differently? This is the power of Pavlov's conditioning, salivating to the bell or any other trigger, and it is how humans are wired to react. Over 80% of your life is running in autopilot, and they run for a lifetime, unless you consciously change them. Once we know how to stop it, we can do something different. You will learn to change your response to the triggers, by stopping them, engaging the higher brain and transferring skills from one situation to another. When you use healthy social defence skills, you won't activate the high arousal system or the reptilian immobiliser.

You are going to practise using your facial expression, your tone of voice, posture, and gestures that you would use when you are expressing yourself like an adult ("do you want a cup of tea?", or "no, I don't want a biscuit"). Remember, the muscles in the face, middle ear, larynx and your tone of voice change your physiology because they are attached to the healthy system, so make sure you're using all the healthy nonverbal signals for each resource.

I spent my life not wanting to be triggered by other people's anger, dominance or criticism but didn't know how to quickly stop the autopilot and access resourcefulness, until I learnt the neuro-linguistic programming (NLP) technique of associating into healthy states. If any of this resonates with you, then look at the online videos showing how to use the Traffic Lights technique and associate into healthy states at www.resettothrive.co.uk. You can learn how to stop old habits, which you hate, and which limit you, and learn how to feel assertive, confident, express yourself and deal with any challenges. One of the greatest gifts of being human is to have a voice, so learn to use it. I call it showing up, letting the world see and hear you, just like everything else in nature. If you have too much anger in your voice, take responsibility, become more reasonable in expressing yourself and check out where so much anger is coming from. We are all looking to become more balanced, finding the middle way, more resourceful.

The lady in the example above had used the Traffic Lights procedure so regularly that it had become much easier for her to switch from an unhealthier state to a healthy, robust state. She wasn't in autopilot yet with the healthy responses, so had to go off to the loo to do a manual reset, then proceed. In the beginning, it is very useful to follow the Traffic Lights procedure exactly as taught. Eventually, with regular use, you will no longer be conditioned to respond inappropriately to triggers and will automatically respond appropriately.

Never berate yourself for needing to skill up; very few people were ever taught social defence skills or emotional literacy when they were growing up, and many weren't allowed to use them. Most people struggle to communicate effectively in every situation, whether they have had CFS or not, and adult relations can be tricky, because we went into adulthood, equipped only with skills from childhood. Like parenting, we are just thrown into adulting with the skills we acquired as children, and then we all just muddle through! Few people are taught the resources for adulting but thankfully today there is more emphasis on social and emotional skills development for youngsters.

Now you have a great opportunity to acquire the resources needed to stay healthy and be robust, even when there are challenges. A caveat of course is never to use these techniques to get yourself into a healthy state for dealing with persistent situations. If the unhealthy person or unhealthy situation persists, even though you use robust social defence skills, then the chimp and reptile will kick in to defend you. It is not healthy to stay in that chronic, unhealthy environment, and so finding a healthy environment is essential.

Symbols and Conditioning

Get into the habit of bringing up symbols, like the bell meaning food for a dog, or a ping alert making you respond to your mobile phone. As you become conditioned to respond to symbols, you will automatically elicit the state you associate with them. I bring up:

- A pink rose for confidence.
- A sword for courage, running down my spine, the handles across my shoulder blades, staying upright and robust.
- My newborn babies, for unconditional love; feeling good about myself, and knowing that life does not have to be perfect to be wonderful.
- A cup of tea for being able to talk easily and openly, even with challenging conversations.
- A Christmas card that wasn't posted, to remind me of my dignity.

Before, you had little choice in how you were shaped, but now you can choose how you want to respond, no matter what the circumstance.

By bringing up a memory, you are also accessing the feeling and the physiology associated with that moment. Your brain has hardwired every memory, every experience, with a physiological response; this is how the amygdala knows to attach fear to certain scenarios. Now, choose healthy reactions instead, and feel how empowering it is.

When you practise this enough, you will be amazed how you can be unaffected by situations that you used to find hard. When you use Traffic Lights to stop being physically aroused by specific triggers, tones of voice or facial expressions, you can respond as the clearheaded, intelligent you. Go online at www.resettothrive.co.uk and see how clients use techniques to access different healthy states.

Having a say in how you do life is such a valuable part of being human. Remember when you were a child and wanted to grow up because "adults get to do what they want, and children have to do as they are told"? Well, now, using the TL technique, you can access what it is to be an adult and decide what you want and how you want to be. Millions of people become grown-ups, without feeling like adults a lot of the time, just because they didn't know how to access the skills that are needed for healthy adulting.

If you come across people who carry on bullying or treat you inappropriately, even though you have used powerful assertive strategies with them, you may need to leave the situation, tell them to leave, or seek professional help. If it is your boss, you may need to take the situation higher up the chain, enlist professional support or ultimately, leave a toxic environment. It is amazing though how often situations can be resolved when you add defence skills to your already competent social skills set.

Summary

- There may be some genetic predisposition influencing a susceptibility to arousal and to ultimately having the reptile kick in. Individual differences in physiology may make you more susceptible to having a dysfunctional autonomic nervous system and CFS. This may explain why some people get overloaded but don't have the reptile kicking in to shut down the body. Instead, they may be more prone to heart, gut, migraine, mental health issues or immune diseases. Whatever the pre-requisites, you can recover and be healthy.
- Porges has shown that there are three levels of defence and human social skills should be our first line of defence in

conflict. They should be used all the time so that we remain in a calm, healthy parasympathetic state. We should only use the mammalian chimp defence or the reptile as a last resort, such as a life-threatening event.

- People with CFS may lack the first line of defence, and therefore only have mammalian and reptilian defences, which are far too powerful for regular use. They became the default mode in many situations, hence the malfunctioning neurological condition for CFS and most symptoms with Long Covid.

- People who do not use the first line of defence may not have learnt the skills growing up or were forbidden from answering back. However, you will struggle in adult relationships if the human defence skills are missing or ineffective. Thus, the inappropriate use of the chimp and the reptile continues into adult life.

- If you live with chronic and persistent dysfunctional behaviour, at work or home, social skills will be insufficient; level 2, fight and flight will be activated automatically and if this doesn't resolve the problem, the reptile will shut down the body to protect it from further onslaught.

- Other peoples' tone of voice, facial expression, posture and gestures trigger a physiological response in us, putting us into thrive or survive modes. (Porges 2001). Friendly faces and gentle tones sooth and nurture us. If people sound scary or dominant, it doesn't mean they are a threat. Mindfulness is a good exercise for developing this recognition. Retrain the amygdala so that nothing is actually scary; you don't need protection.

- Any healthy adult can still develop unhealthy responses if they live in harsh conditions. If they are naturally caring, kind and generous, they may show care, empathy and understanding, even when it is misplaced because in doing so, they maintain unhealthy relationships. Most youngsters in nurturing families learn to be compliant to reasonable demands, but these same people often continue to comply, even when it isn't appropriate later in life, when they live or work with tigers.

- We need to increase the tools in our toolbox, be more resourceful and have greater flexibility in dealing with everything and everyone, by using the Traffic Lights procedure and associating into healthy states. When we become more resourceful, we increase our supplies and can meet demands better. As we bridge the gap between supply and demands, there is no need to activate the turbo charge defences. Become mindfully aware of your triggers and your response.

- Review all your patterns that were inappropriately causing you to fire off the chimp or reptile too much. Learn to set boundaries and know your limitations as a human; you are not God.

- Most people, including those who had CFS, have excellent social skills for engaging, caring and empathy but now they need to add defence and protective skills to their toolbox and have a more robust skill set.

- Use the Traffic Lights procedure to step into what it feels like to be resourceful, accessing whichever skill is needed for each occasion and practise the healthy responses.

- Everyone has all the resources they need; it is just that they weren't triggered in certain scenarios. Transfer skills, from when you can use them naturally, to moments when they were inhibited by triggers, using TL. Everything is about balance and deciding if a particular response is appropriate in a particular situation.

- Empathy, kindness, and support are appropriate when the other person is not harming you, overloading you or draining you. Protective skills include saying no, having healthy boundaries, and being self-assured. Learn to express yourself easily, openly, to have a voice and be assertive. Show up as an equal, because you matter as much as any other person, not more than or less than.

- If the defence social skills are not sufficient for resolving conflict and discord, ask the other person to leave or, if it is your boss, take it higher, but stay strong and robust. If all else fails, leave the unhealthy environment.

- Any habit needs lots of practise and repetition before it is automatic, so be prepared to commit to becoming healthier and having healthy responses. Think how many times you had to practise before you were proficient at other skills, driving, sports, work skills. Be prepared to have old habits pop up intermittently or triggered by PIES overload; do not be shocked, just do the work to stop them until they are permanently extinguished. Use your resourceful tools to stay in the parasympathetic system.

- Access the FEARLESS tools using the Traffic Lights procedure. This should be how you approach life in future. Continue to use your BETTER exercises, to activate the body, and ensure you have restorative sleep.

Life is precious. Wouldn't it be great to do it the very best way we can? Choose a healthy habitat, surrounded by nurturing supportive people. Use your Traffic Lights procedure to access healthy resources and access the times when you have the defence skills. You can choose when it is appropriate to use your empathy and caring skills and when it is more appropriate to employ healthy, protective defence skills. When you have all the tools in your toolbox, you will stay healthy, no matter what life throws at you, as long as your environment is nurturing.

This is the key to health. Develop a buffer against harsh conditions by learning defence skills. When you use level 1 defences all the time, you will not rouse the chimp or the reptile, and therefore, you will not have a malfunctioning neurological condition like CFS ever again.

Chapter 9:
A Bright Future

"A bright future beckons. The onus is on us, through hard work, honesty and integrity, to reach for the stars." - Nelson Mandela

Take yourself forward five years, seeing yourself up there on a screen and notice how healthy you are, with your human defence armour protecting you from demands and challenges. Bring up all the symbols you associate with health and FEARLESS living and step into that healthy you, the one who is so well rehearsed in being strong, robust, and fearless. Step into that new you and feel what it feels like, living this way, easily and effortlessly.

What to do with Viruses in Future

Since the amygdala records an emotion for every experience we have ever had, there is a good chance that the brain will have lodged viruses as scary and associate them with chronic fatigue syndrome (CFS), Long Covid fatigue. It is normal and understandable that we feel scared at the thought of being stuck with post viral fatigue, Long Covid or CFS again when we get a virus in future, but it is not useful. So much of my follow-up support with clients was dealing with their response to viruses. Here is a typical reaction to viruses or infections returning:

> *Meg regularly phoned when she had a sore throat, in a panic. "My chronic fatigue started with a sore throat from an infection; I'm so scared it's coming back". Clearly, the unconscious brain has made the association that "a virus means CFS" so, being the vigilant brain that it is, it alerts her to danger and protects her, either by putting her into high arousal for fight and flight or by immobilising her. In survival mode, the anti-inflammatory system couldn't function, so the pain got worse, the glands swelled up and in the end, she became trapped in the perpetuating cycle, getting stuck.*

You are probably aware by now that it was not the sore throat that caused her body to pack in so dramatically with CFS, it was just the straw that broke the camel's back. In Meg's case, she had been completing a Master's degree whilst working as an orthoptist, which led her to burn the candle at both ends. She was also anxious about her exams and had been dealing with a difficult boss. As symptoms returned now, she needed to remind herself that the sore throat she is experiencing is just a sore throat, and it wasn't the thing that created her downfall.

Bizarrely, when I speak with Meg, I get a sore throat, even though I don't suffer from sore throats - that's the power of the brain. That's empathy. We laugh about my sore throat, and I ask her, what would she advise me to do to get rid of it? She replies: "It will pass, focus on something else, take paracetamol and see the GP if it doesn't settle. You won't get CFS back." Suddenly her belief has changed, her perception of reality has shifted to feeling safe, and she is laughing. She took her own advice and of course recovered.

Beliefs and perception can very easily get you stuck. If you believe you can't recover and believe symptoms are scary, then you will turn off all the systems needed to heal the body and recover from viruses. If you believe you will not get over the virus this time, symptoms will be prolonged because you are not doing the work, and you will go into a downward spiral.

When you have had a bad experience with viruses, and the brain has hardwired the idea that "viruses means fatigue again", don't be alarmed. It simply learnt something new about viruses and it is your job to retrain the brain that you know how to deal with viruses, and you *are* safe. You do not need the protective brain kicking in.

I still have moments when I haven't recovered after a couple of days and worry, "I should have recovered by now", or feel concerned if my symptoms recur. Then I do the Traffic Light procedure to regain my confidence and do recovery the right way. We started the journey to recovery with a chapter on beliefs because beliefs are so powerful, and beliefs will change when you have had a bad experience. It is up to all of us to stay focused and nurture healthy beliefs.

It is essential to stop this association between viruses and getting ill again. Be confident that a virus will not result in CFS, Long Covid fatigue or PVFS. Besides, you are going to change how you respond to life and keep yourself healthy. If the brain learnt that viruses are scary, you need to retrain it back to healthy associations with infections; people get them and recover. Tell the amygdala:

> *"I know how to deal with viruses now; I am going to rest, and rest assured I will get over this virus. I am going to treat myself as I would another person, with care and compassion, and I will be fine. I don't need protecting because I've got this. I can do this, and I do not need the protective brain taking over, thank you."*

You must shift beliefs about viruses, and if the unhealthy thoughts come back, you need to give yourself a good talking to (with compassion) and use your Traffic Lights to access FEARLESS recovery resources. Then cheer! Be proud that you have overcome this. Very few people realise that eighty percent of everything we do in life is a conditioned response to everything around us, so it is hardly surprising that a virus triggered fear when we had bad experiences with them before. The brain learnt it was scary, and it would have carried on responding like that forever, but you took control and stopped it! Give yourself a massive pat on the back, smile, whoop, because you have just had a Battle of the Brains and the higher, conscious brain is back on top. Hurrah!

EXERCISE. Sit in a quiet spot or lie down, whatever is comfortable for you. Take yourself back to a time when you were a child, and you recovered from any illness, a cold, tummy bug, sore throat, anything. You can feel what it feels like being that child, milking it for all it's worth, getting days off school and treats and attention. You took it for granted you would recover. Take in what you are seeing, hearing, and doing as you know this, and notice how everyone around you knows that you will soon recover. With this in mind, feel what it feels like again to relax.

When you remember what it was like to take it for granted again, open your eyes, and laugh at yourself for having a wobble and for sorting it. With your healthy, normal belief, do the work to recover. You can use the Traffic Lights procedure to stop any panic or concern, to engage the rational brain and then step into you as a child, taking it for granted you will recover. Walk the Talk.

Go back through your recovery programme, doing FEARLESS resources, and using TL to access these resources if you are having any wobbles during recovery from viruses in the future. As you lie in bed, letting the body use its energy reserves for dealing with the virus, use your BETTER vagal exercises to stay in the healthy vagal system: breathing, meditations, chanting, humming, singing, and gargling. Focus on getting better and not on all the jobs you "have to do". Better to fully recover than to go back on a low threshold, then suffer again. Most people will have setbacks when recovering from any virus, but they will often rightfully assume they will get better. There is an exercise online, used by respiratory physiotherapists, at www.resettothrive.co.uk, which shows you how to breathe, if you are struggling with a respiratory infection; it is crucial to stay calm, as shallow breathing will activate the sympathetic system, and you want to counterbalance this reflex reaction, not exacerbate it.

Complete Recovery

Finally, many people seem to think that they can get better, but never be one hundred percent better after long term illnesses. It is interesting that they believe they can do the work to get ninety-five percent better, but that the same tools don't work for the last, tiny bit. That doesn't make sense. They believe it isn't possible to fully recover and have become conditioned to be cautious. It is absolutely not true that we can't fully recover. If you notice yourself doing this, stop the perpetuating cycle, laugh at yourself, and do your Traffic Lights to regain confidence and trust in yourself and in life again. You always took it for granted you could do life before and you can take it for granted again when you have healthy beliefs and do the work. Then, when you feel good, do something a little bit extra to prove to yourself, and the protective brain, that you can.

You should expect to be able to do whatever someone of your age group can do and what was normal before. My clients and I live normal healthy lives, walking, cycling, working, dancing, doing sports, and whatever we want to do. If you believe you became ill because you did too much and you fear hitting the tolerance level again, you will live a half-life. Stop. You have learnt that it is important to live in a healthy environment, you have developed robust defence skills and can set healthy boundaries with people and tasks. You are robust and skilled; you are not going to be automatically triggered into old patterns, and you can take control of demands by working out what you value, what matters, and dump anything that is not essential. You will know how to deal with viruses in the future, no matter how powerful they are.

It is possible to be triggered back into symptoms a long time after you have recovered, because once the brain has learnt a habit, it can pop up for some time until it is fully extinguished. Expect it and do not be surprised or devastated. The Traffic Lights procedure is so handy; if you notice anything coming back, stop it, and get yourself working again. You can then consider if anything triggered this, or whether you have been pushing through, being unreasonable.

For me, after recovering, emotional and social load from life events was a trigger, and I had to do TL to limit their impact. Emotions are healthy but not in excess. I used the Traffic Lights to get my body working, and then engaged rational thinking to resolve the problem or let it go, depending on the problem. Sports people are trained to let go of failures and upsets; their mantra is "park it, move on " and we can do that too. Also, I still reacted inappropriately to viruses for many years, and had to do the work, every time, to get back on track. As Nelson Mandela said, "don't judge me by my successes, judge me by how many times I fell down and got back up again." Absolutely! Resilience is key.

Be the bouncy ball and decide to get back up again.

In the early days of permanent recovery, I still had to be mindful of my enthusiast pattern; I still did too much and kept going too long without stopping, even though the body was straining and needed a break. I was certainly not living a cautious life or keeping safe within a low threshold; my activities levels were still unrealistic and abnormal. I would do a full-time job, work in the evenings with clients, and then renovate my house till midnight or beyond, a pattern I kept up for years. Finally, I had to commit to having a better balance between working and having breaks, so I learnt the art of relaxation, having to consciously listen to my body and be aware of my patterns. I hadn't practised the art of relaxing for many years, so it was a conscious effort to make the change, just as it is with any habit. When you go beyond human capacity, something has to give, and it cannot be your body ever again.

Learn to:

- Become mindful of patterns that are not useful and commit to becoming better.
- Do the Traffic Lights procedure any time your body needs a manual override. Never use Traffic Lights to keep going with unreasonable demands.
- Have a healthy balanced lifestyle and environment.
- Use your defence skills to stay in the parasympathetic mode, regardless of what challenges life throws at you.
- Change your beliefs and perception of life. Nothing matters more than having health for you and your loved ones. Nothing is a tiger, so don't activate ancient defences.
- Care less about the things you used to care too much about.
- Change the things you can change and have the serenity to accept the things you can't.
- Put in the effort, giving time and commitment to things you value most - your health and wellbeing included.

When you do this, the symptoms stop permanently. There is no magic, only the wisdom to know what is happening to your body, why it is happening, and then it is up to you to do the work and make it healthy again. The body is a miracle, life is a miracle, and we are so fortunate that this condition can be corrected. This approach won't cure damaged organs, but we can reset the malfunctioning system that is causing so many symptoms.

You have a job to do, so treat it like any job; just get on with what you need to do. Naturally, you will be shocked and even frightened or terrified initially, but within a few minutes, take the reins and do the work, calmly and confidently, using all your FEARLESS tools.

Keep doing BETTER practises to activate the vagal system and stay healthy, including having restorative sleep. Vagal exercises, including yoga and meditation are essential but not sufficient; they are the posts on the fence of life. We need to live our lives consistently consciously, mindfully, detached from anything that doesn't serve us and make our environment more nurturing. Use your Traffic Lights to maintain the healthy track and access healthy responses. Always go back to your summaries, the videos, the book, and your journal to remind yourself what to do, because as we said, anything you learn will be forgotten unless you refresh yourself.

For over fourteen years now, I have been fully fit, had no symptoms and do whatever I like. I am no longer affected by other people or things; nothing and nobody will ever wake the reptile again. Thousands of people do fully recover. So can you.

I don't like the idea that recovery has to be lightning quick, or that you can go to a practitioner who waves a magic wand and makes you feel fully better. I believe it does work for those who are *already* masters of FEARLESS, who are well rehearsed in being completely focused on the task, and switch their perception of things quickly, calmly and apply those skills to recovery. However, other people who believe they should recover quickly and then receive symptoms again often assume they have failed, that there is something seriously wrong with them, that the programme didn't work or that "you can't really recover from CFS and Long Covid". All these scenarios get you stuck, or mean you give up. Many people resign themselves to having it forever after they have had a relapse or symptoms return. Please, do not do that. Become brilliant at your FEARLESS resources, do your BETTER exercises and then, and only then, do the quick technique of associating into states, intentionally provided at the end of Part One on recovery.

You can very quickly recover, but like an aeroplane leaving a residual trail, there will be things you will still need to work on, including improving your skill set, how you do life, and making conditions for yourself better. When my clients come to me, they can feel healthy very quickly, but they know they have been given the tools to do the work if and when anything pops back. Life will always throw us curve balls and viruses.

Commit to the tools you have been given in the book and if you need a further shift, enlist the support of practitioners, therapists, or coaches to keep you motivated and committed to change. People seem happy to commit time and money on cosmetic changes or hobbies. Surely it is worth investing time and effort into changing patterns that don't serve you well in life, either for your health or in relationships. Even if you find a particularly entrenched pattern, that's okay, because you have a little tool in your back pocket - the Traffic Lights procedure with the NLP technique of stepping into better states - to do a manual override and then proceed. Some patterns may need a manual override for years and others for less time, but it is worth it to have a better life. I still do a manual override sometimes on automatic patterns and then get back on track, responding in a more useful way. How lovely to have a Traffic Lights tool to quickly reset to thrive. If your patterns are still entrenched, do consider EMDR or a similar support, because your health and wellbeing are treasures worth looking after.

Remember:

Focus. Focus on what you want, NOT on the things you don't want.

Effort. Put in the effort and do the work.

Effortless. This is when you are back running in autopilot, not having to do a manual override.

Determined. Be determined to do what it takes, no matter how long it takes or how many times you need to do it, until you achieve your goal. When you truly want to be better, do the work and be empowered. When you have been running patterns in autopilot for a long time, it would be reasonable to expect that you will need to practise the new pathways, a lot, for them to become the autopilot. Do a manual reset with Traffic Lights until you go into autopilot and begin to respond automatically.

Even if symptoms pop back long after you thought you had fully recovered, stop, take control, do your Traffic Lights and associate into a healthy body. You can get the body working again and keep doing it until the reptile stops coming to the rescue and the circuit is extinguished forever.

I would urge everyone to use and practise their defence social skills; setting boundaries, speaking up, showing up, because then you are robust and capable of doing this life, no matter what curve balls it throws at you. When you use your first line of defence and have a healthy armour to ward off overload and conflict, you are not turning on the ancient circuits to engage the chimp and the reptile. You can't have a malfunctioning autonomic system when it is being used properly, therefore, you won't get symptoms associated with survival responses. The gut, immune system and metabolic systems can then rebalance. I suggest, to be fully healthy, you find a deep sense of everything being okay. Use your Traffic Lights to access this feeling and reconnect life with the vagal system.

If you ever notice yourself going into any of the stages of arousal, resistance and illness talked about in the general adaptive syndrome (Selye, 1936), then stop and work out what you need to do instead. Use your Traffic Lights to access clear headed problem solving, then consider where you are going off track. Are you always using your FEARLESS resources? Is there overload again, harsh conditions, problems that need resolving, are you using your human defence skills adequately or using the chimp again? Have you fallen back into old habits like I did? Are you using Traffic Lights to access states you need; assertiveness, problem solving, letting go, or whatever you need to stay in the green track?

Enthusiasts will need to check with other people what they think is a reasonable amount to take on. It is easy to say yes to projects, because from a distance they seem easy and manageable. For instance, it is normal to be excited about applying for a job but as reality looms, we can be a bit anxious about what we have agreed to take on, and how we are going to fit it in. Enthusiasts just seem to do this to a greater degree than other people, unaware in their enthusiasm that they are biting off more than they can chew. Again, there is nothing wrong with any pattern, as long as it isn't excessive, because the body loves moderation and balance. Remember to keep a note of how long you think it will take and how long it actually takes. You are looking to lead a full life, not a crazy life. Listen to people's comments and notice if they think you never stop or wonder how you keep going. Ask people to check out if what you are doing is reasonable. If people say you should take a break, then they are probably right. You may notice you get absorbed in something and can carry on for hours, so challenge this pattern. There is a happy balance. Become fascinated by people who are healthy and how much they can relax, sleep and chill. Learn the art of doing nothing and feeling guilt free about it.

If you notice anything getting in your way, look at the video on saboteurs and commit to seeing a practitioner to help shift unconscious patterns, such as an Eye Movement Desensitisation and Reprocessing practitioner (EMDR), counsellor, or an NLP trainer. If you continue to live in harsh, unfavourable conditions, your body *will* struggle to thrive, and doing Traffic Lights to get into healthy states within these environments is like putting a sticky plaster on a wide-open wound. It is a temporary strategy until you can live in more nurturing conditions. Focus on what a healthy habitat means for you.

Ultimately, for me, the gift of life is the most precious gift we have been given. To live well is to maintain our spirit, no matter how many curveballs life throws at us. Life is not a mechanical, cold entity: it is the wonder of nature, a smile, laughter, joy, kindness, sharing and love. If you have lost your spirit, if you have lost your sparkle, then the greatest gift, once you fully recover, is to go on a quest to get it back again and have fun doing it.

In human development we talk about the spiritual aspect of life, that part of you that rises above the struggling human mode, connecting with a much higher, greater perspective that enables us to let go of the things we thought mattered and rise above our human state. PIES becomes SPIES as we include this additional Spiritual dimension. In his book, *Why God Won't Go Away: Brain Science and the Biology of Belief* (2002), Dr Andrew Newberg explains how we are neurologically programmed as humans to access higher states. When we sing, chant, do repetitive movement, prayer and connect with nature, we fire off the parts of the brain that give us a deep sense of belonging, connection, and fulfilment. So, shake your booty, sing, chant, hum, and connect with nature again to access the greatest level of health and wellbeing. It is also useful to step into a metaphor of what it is to be spiritual, strong and serene by borrowing from nature. We are deeply connected to nature and can imagine what it feels like to be as free as the wind, as stable and grounded as the trees, or as powerful as the sea, because we are part of nature, programmed to be spiritual and to understand symbolism. Words, art, letters, represent something meaningful to us. Use the metaphor on the green part of the Traffic Lights procedure; it is particularly useful for people who feel it is so long ago that they had a good moment, or who pollute great moments with negative memories.

For me, the spiritual aspect was essential for recovery. When I was bedridden, it was an absolute game changer to be able to rise above my struggling human state and give it all up to a higher energy and by stepping into metaphors of wellbeing from nature. By feeling in awe of the wonder and power of nature, it allowed my body to settle back into the healthy parasympathetic state. Once I could move again, being in nature became my medicine. I would at first just sit in my small garden, but when I was finally able to, I walked the country lanes and the sand dunes at Northam Burrows, looking out to the sea and singing uplifting songs as I walked. Call on the power of nature, the power of our miraculous human brain with its capacity to access higher, healthy states, anytime you need it. I am sure that accessing this spiritual or higher consciousness was the difference between me being stuck, terrified in bed, and eventually being able to move again.

Become FEARLESS and access all the states you need to thrive. The journey to recovery from Long Covid and CFS has been hard, and it has taken great effort, but you can come out of this better, stronger, and more resilient than before, ready to enjoy this wonderful world and stay healthy. Be so proud of yourself for conquering a challenge as big as Mount Everest. You are amazing. Celebrate and be excited!

If you can do that, you can do anything.

In A Nutshell

- Chronic fatigue syndrome (CFS) and for many people with Long Covid, is a breakdown of the autonomic nervous system, and a malfunctioning neurological illness. When the survival system has become the dominant mode, your body will feel the effects; at least 20 metabolic functions slow down as you are put into tick over mode, which keeps you stationary but safe. The body had been bombarded and had enough; it had gone beyond the healthy threshold, which led to shut down.

- The body is designed to Thrive or Survive. In unfavourable environments, it is put into survival mode. Attack from physical and psychological environmental factors changes the body at a cellular level. Healing proceeds only once the body gets the "all clear" signal that it is safe to recover, otherwise it gets stuck in a loop, causing sickness behaviours and symptoms. To thrive, you need to be telling your amygdala, your lookout (which we refer to as the meerkat throughout the book), that you are safe in this world, *even if* you have symptoms. You need to let it know that, even if you cannot do everything yet, that stairs, activity, and mobilising are in themselves not dangerous. They are neutral events and objects. It needs signs that you are capable, any green shoots of recovery, to register you don't need protecting.

- The Sympathetic Nervous System (SNS) and dorsal nerve are our ancient survival systems. SNS is the mammalian system designed for fight and flight, to mobilise you and put you into arousal and get you out of danger. The dorsal is an ancient relic, reptilian mode, making the body freeze. It shuts down the body and is only used as a last resort or if you experienced a trauma. With CFS and Long Covid fatigue, when your body feels over aroused, it is in SNS. When your body has shut down, it is in reptilian mode, ticking over. Safe but immobilised.

- Your amygdala has learnt that life with CFS or similar illnesses is scary and that the symptoms are scary, so it is telling the body to *stay* in survival mode as a way to protect you from harm. This creates a vicious cycle. It also becomes a conditioned response as you were initially exposed to activity or events with too low a threshold; then, whenever you are exposed to those triggers in future, the body will automatically react to it because it doesn't want you to do anything it now "knows" is a threat. It will throw you into arousal, pain, tension, nausea, brain fog, or shut you down. Your survival system has now been hardwired to outside stimuli, just like Pavlov's dogs' salivary glands became hardwired to the sound of a bell. You have to let the protective brain know that nothing is scary, that you can deal with this, and stay calm. That will hardwire neutral events back onto the healthy branch, our vagal system, that lets the body thrive.

- If you believe you can, or believe you can't, you are absolutely right. We can find evidence to justify all our beliefs but that doesn't mean they are true. Terrorists, warmongers, and dictators can all spout evidence supporting their belief and their cause. Evidence doesn't mean their belief is healthy. Believe you can recover because thousands of people do. There are some interesting and unhealthy beliefs out there from professionals, support associations and activists. They have the right to believe whatever they like and whatever serves them; you have the right to choose whichever belief you know is healthy for recovery. Believe what resonates with you and what serves you, what is useful for you. Beliefs get you stuck, so be aware of any limiting beliefs you hold, both during your recovery and when you are fit again.

To recover, we need to turn on the thrive mode, the healthy parasympathetic system, and turn off our survival systems. To do this we need to perceive the world is a safe place and tell the amygdala you are safe, even if you are ill and on your journey to recovery. You will stop all fear, anxiety, and concerns about being immobilised and shut down because fear fires off the survival system that is already running amok. Instead, you will activate FEARLESS resources, consistently, that activate the healthy vagal nerve, which is part of your parasympathetic system. These are:

- Focus on signs of recovery, so the brain registers health and that you can do life safely.
- Excited and enthusiastic. Activate healthy chemicals, like endorphins, that are essential for healing.
- Adapt: the body will naturally adapt back to the healthy state when the environment is nurturing. Make it nurturing, manageable, and let the protective brain know you are safe in this world, even though you have symptoms and / or are bedridden.
- Resilient. Whenever you fall down or have setbacks, pick yourself up and try again.

- Love. The greatest healing hormone is oxytocin, so fire it off by being kind and compassionate to yourself, and have loving, nurturing people to support you, if possible. Remove yourself from hostility and blame, internally and from others, because that cannot serve you.
- Emotionally detached. Become a mindful observer of anything that doesn't serve you. Simply notice symptoms and other people's expressions from a place of detachment and curiosity.
- Serenity. Learn amazing grace and peaceful courage because you will need it to reactivate the calm parasympathetic system, which is designed to heal and repair the body.
- See Things Differently. As you practice mindfulness, simply notice that symptoms are just sensations. Hostile faces or an angry tone of voice are just muscles moving and sounds being expressed. Imagine nausea turning into clowns tumbling, or however you want to see them, a safe and harmless association. Again, this makes your brain detect a nurturing environment, so the body can naturally revert to thrive.

Do your BETTER vagal exercises to activate the vagus nerve in your larynx, throat, lungs, heart, gut and all the organs in the immune system. These exercises include breathing from your diaphragm, singing, chanting, gargling, cold showers, or cold-water swimming. Do exercises and activities that you enjoy, engaging your body, one step at a time. Do your Traffic Lights to stop inappropriate responses and consciously do a manual override to reset to thrive mode. Restorative rest and sleep are your body's natural repair system, so prioritise doing the guidance to reset the circadian cycle. Getting agitated or anxious when you lie down only perpetuates the malfunctioning system. Restorative rest requires you to be lying at ease and relaxed. May you enjoy and be grateful for this incredible, miraculous gift of life, and doing it the right way.

DON'T JUST SURVIVE - RESET TO THRIVE!

References

Ader, Robert, Felten, David L. & Cohen, Nicholas. (1991). *Psychoneuroimmunology, Second Edition -1991*. Academic Press.

Barlow, C., Walklate, S., Johnson, K., Humphreys, L. and Kirby, S. (2018) *Police responses to coercive control*. Published online: N8 Policing Research Partnership

Bamforth, N. (1993) *M.E. (Chronic Fatigue Syndrome) and the Healer Within*. Oxford, UK. Amethyst Books.

Ben Hunt-Davis, B. and Beveridge, H. (2011) *Will It Make The Boat Go Faster?* Leicester UK. Matador.

Bolte Taylor, J. PhD. (2008) *My Stroke of Insight*. London. Hodder and Stoughton.

Bowlby, J. and Ainsworth, M. (1992). "The origins of attachment theory". *Developmental Psychology* 28, pp. 759-775. Routledge.

Brenner, H. and Schöttker, B., (2020). Vitamin D insufficiency may account for almost ninc of ten COVID-19 deaths. Time to act. comment on: "Vitamin D deficiency and outcome of COVID-19 patients". nutrients 2020, 12, 2757. *Nutrients*, 12(12), p.3642. https://doi.org/10.3390/nu12123642

Buczynski, R. PhD and Porges, S. PhD. (2014) Transcript of: "How Polyvagal Theory Expands Our Healing Paradigm". www.nicabm.com

Buczynski, R. PhD and Porges, S. PhD. (2015) Transcript of: "Polyvagal Theory Can Revolutionize Your Work with Trauma Survivors". www.nicabm.com

Chinagudi, S., *et al*. (2014) "Immediate effect of short duration of slow deep breathing on heart rate variability in healthy adults". *National Journal of Physiology, Pharmacy and Pharmacology* 4(3), pp. 233-235 Abstract.

Cleare, A. J. (2004) "The HPA axis and the genesis of chronic fatigue syndrome". *Trends in Endocrinology & Metabolism*, 15(2), p. 55-59. Abstract. https://doi.org/10.1016/j.tem.2003.12.002.

Cohen, S., Tyrrell, D.A., and Smith, A.P. (1991) "Psychological stress and susceptibility to the common cold" *New England journal of medicine*, 325(9), pp. 606-612.

Costeira, R. and Lee, K. Dr. (2020) "Post-menopausal women at higher risk of developing severe COVID-19". *medRxiv*. https://www.kcl.ac.uk/news/post-menopausal-women-higher-risk-developing-severe-covid-19

Dana, D., (2018) *The Polyvagal theory in therapy: engaging the rhythm of regulation* (Norton series on interpersonal neurobiology). New York. WW Norton and Company.

Dunbar, R., (2021) *Friends: Understanding the Power of Our Most Important Relationships*. London. Little Brown.

Freeman, R. and Komaroff, A. L., (1997). "Does the chronic fatigue syndrome involve the autonomic nervous system?". *The American Journal of Medicine*, 102 (4), pp. 357-364. https://doi.org/10.1016/S0002-9343(97)00087-9

Garner, P., (2021) "Long-haul COVID brings long road to recovery". *WebMD*. https://www.webmd.com/lung/news/20210630/long-haul-covid-brings-long-road-to-recovery

Goertzel, B. N. *et al.* (2006) "Allostatic load is associated with symptoms in chronic fatigue syndrome patients". *Future Medicine Ltd*, 7(3), pp. 485-494. https://doi.org/10.2217/14622416.7.3.485

Goertzel, B. N. *et al.* (2006) "Combinations of single nucleotide polymorphisms in neuroendocrine effector and receptor genes predict chronic fatigue syndrome". *Future Medicine Ltd*, 7(3), pp. 475-483. *https://doi.org/10.2217/14622416.7.3.475*

Hall, N., and O'Grady. M. (1991) "Psychosocial interventions and immune function" – *Psychoneuroimmunology (Second edition)*, pp. 1067-1080. New York. Academic Press. https://doi.org/10.1016/B978-0-12-043780-1.50045-2

Hamilton, D. (2008) *It's the Thought that Counts*. London. Hay House Inc.

Hamilton, D. (2008) *How Your Mind Can Heal Your Body*. London. Hay House Inc.

Hanlon, M. (2013) "Scientists Under Siege". The Sunday Times, May 5th, pp12-19.

Harry F. Harlow, H. F. and Zimmerman, R. (1958). "The development of affectional responses in infant monkeys". *Proceedings of the*

American Philosophical Society, 102(5), pp. 501-509

Heijmans, H. (1998) "Coping and adaptive outcome in chronic fatigue syndrome: importance of illness cognitions." *Journal of psychosomatic research* 45 (1), pp. 39-51. https://doi.org/10.1016/S0022-3999(97)00265-1

Holt-Lunstad, J., Smith, T., and Bradley Layton, J. (2010) "Social relationships and mortality risk: a meta-analytic review". *PLOS medicine*, 7(7). p.e1000316 Social Relationships and Mortality Risk: A Meta-analytic Review (plos.org)

Holt-Lunstad, J., 2020. Social isolation and health. *Health affairs brief*. https://www.healthaffairs.org/do/10.1377/hpb20200622.253235/

Kamau-Mitchell, C. (2021) "GPs need awareness about post-covid ME/CFS".bmj, 374

(12th August): n1995 doi: https://doi.org/10.1136/bmj.n1995

Kiecolt-Glaser, J. and Glaser. R. (1991) "Stress and immune function in humans". *Psychoneuroimmunology (Second edition)*, pp. 849-867. Academic Press.

Lipton, B. (2005) *Biology of Belief*. California. Elite Books.

Maloney, E. M *et al.* (2006) "Chronic fatigue syndrome and high allostatic load" *Future Medicine Ltd*, 7(3), pp. 467-473. *https://doi.org/10.2217/14622416.7.3.467*

McEwan, B., and Laslcy, E., (2002) *The End of Stress As We Know It*. New York. Dana Press.

Meltzer, D.O., Best, T.J., Zhang, H., Vokes, T., Arora, V. and Solway, J., 2020. Association of vitamin D deficiency and treatment with COVID-19 incidence. *MedRxiv*. https://doi.org/10.1101/2020.05.08.20095893

Moldofsky, H. (1993) "Fibromyalgia, sleep disorder and chronic fatigue syndrome" *Chronic Fatigue Syndrome* Edited Whelan, J and Bock, G. pp. 262-271. London. Wiley.

Michael Moseley. (2018) "Trust Me, I'm a Doctor", Mental Health Special. BBC 2 www.bbc.co.uk

Naviaux, R.K., (2014). Metabolic features of the cell danger response. *Mitochondrion*, 16, pp.7-17. https://doi.org/10.1016/j.mito.2013.08.006

Naviaux, R. (2020). "Perspective: Cell danger response Biology- The new science that connects environmental health with mitochondria and the rising tide of chronic illness". *Mitochondrion*, 51(3), pp. 40-45. https://www.sciencedirect.com/science/article/pii/S1567724919302922

Naviaux, R. K., *et al.*, (2016) "Metabolic features of chronic fatigue syndrome" –*Proceedings of the National Academy of Sciences.* 113(37), E5472-E5480. www.pnas.org. https://doi.org/10.1073/pnas.1607571113

Newberg, A. (2002) *Why God Won't go Away: Brain Science and the Biology of Belief.* London. Ballantine Books.

Nicholson T. Dr. (2022) "New study identifies 12 key outcomes to assess Long COVID treatments". *Institute of Psychiatry, Psychology and Neuroscience.* https://www.kcl.ac.uk/news/new-study-identifies-12-key-outcomes-to-assess-long-covid-treatments

Office for National Statistics. (2022) "Prevalence of ongoing symptoms following coronavirus (COVID-19) infection in the UK". https://www.ons.gov.uk/peoplepopulationandcommunity/healthandsocialcare/conditionsanddiseases/bulletins/prevalenceofongoingsymptomsf
ollowingcoronaviruscovid19infectionintheuk/7april2022

Office of National Statistics. (2020) "Parenting in Lockdown. Coronavirus and the effects on work-life balance". https://www.ons.gov.uk/peoplepopulationandcommunity/healthandsocialcare/conditionsanddiseases/datasets/parentinginlockdowncoronavirusandtheeffectsonworklifebalance

Papadopoulos, A. and Cleare, A. (2012) "Hypothalamic–pituitary–adrenal axis dysfunction in chronic fatigue syndrome". *Nat Rev Endocrinol* 8 (1), pp. 22-32. https://doi.org/10.1038/nrendo.2011.153.

Patterson, C., *Man Down by Matt Rudd, review- why are men unhappy?*, Sunday Times magazine, 20th September 2020 https://www.thetimes.co.uk/article/man-down-why-men-are-unhappy-and-what-we-can-do-about-it-by-matt-rudd-book-review-nvm2phd2x

Peck, S. M. (1978) *The Road Less Travelled.* London. Arrow.

Pert, C. PhD. (1997) *Molecules of Emotion.* London. Simon and Schuster.

Porges, S. W. (2001) The polyvagal theory: phylogenetic substrates of a social nervous system. *International journal of psychophysiology,* 42(2), pp.123-146. Elsevier. https://doi.org/10.1016/S0167-8760(01)00162-3

Porges S. (2011) *The Polyvagal Theory: Neurophysiological Foundations of Emotion, Attachment, Communication, and Self-Regulation.* New York. W.W Norton

Reeve, S. (2019) *Step By Step*. London. Hodder and Stoughton.

Rudd, M. (2020) *Man Down: Why Men Are Unhappy and What We Can Do About It*. UK. Piatkus.

Sapolsky, R. M. (2004) *Why Zebras Don't Get Ulcers*.The acclaimed guide to stress,stress related diseases and coping New York. Holt paperbacks.

Sapra, A., Bhandari, P., (2021) Chronic Fatigue Syndrome. Sep 18. In: StatPearls [Internet]. Treasure Island (FL): StatPearls Publishing; 2022 Jan–. PMID: 32491608 https://www.ncbi.nlm.nih.gov/books/NBK557676/

Schonkoff, J. (2017) One million neural connections per second" Center of the DevelopingChild, (https://developingchild.harvard.edu/science/key-concepts/brain-architecture/

Schreiner, P. *et al.* (2020). "Human herpesvirus-6 reactivation, mitochondrial fragmentation, and the coordination of antiviral and metabolic phenotypes in Myalgic encephalomyelitis/chronic fatigue syndrome". *Immunohorizons*, 4 (4), pp. 201-215.

Selye, H. (1936) "A Syndrome Produced by Diverse Noctuous Agents". *Nature 138*, p.32.

Shattuck, E.C. and Muehlenbein, M.P., (2015). Human sickness behavior: Ultimate and proximate explanations. *American Journal of Physical Anthropology*, 157(1), pp.1-18.

Vogt, H., Ulvestad, E., and Bruun Wyller, V., (2016). "Metabolic features of chronic fatigue syndrome revisited". *National Academy of Sciences*, 113(46), pp. E7140-E7141. https://www.pnas.org/doi/full/10.1073/pnas.1615143113

Wong, T. L. and Weitzer, D. J. (2021) "Long COVID and Myalgic Encephalomyelitis/Chronic Fatigue Syndrome (ME/CFS)—A Systematic Review and Comparison of Clinical Presentation and Symptomatology. *Medicina* , 57(5), 418. https://doi.org/10.3390/medicina57050418

World Health Organization, 2021. *A clinical case definition of post COVID-19 condition by a Delphi consensus, 6 October 2021* (No. WHO/2019-nCoV/Post_COVID-19_condition/Clinical_case_definition/2021.1). World Health Organization.

Wyller, V., Eriksen, H.R. and Malterud, K., (2009) "Can sustained arousal explain the Chronic Fatigue Syndrome?". *Behavioural and Brain Functions* 5(1), pp. 1-10.

https://pubmed.ncbi.nlm.nih.gov/19236717/

Wu, Z. and McGoogan, J.M. (2021) "Characteristics of and Important Lessons from the Coronavirus Disease 2019 (Covid-19) outbreak in China".

Online References

www.resettothrive.co.uk

www.ukbiobank.ac.uk

www.nhs.uk (Vit D 400 units per day)

https://english.emmaclit.com/2017/05/20/you-shouldve-asked/

Helen Petersen, "How Millennials became the burnt-out generation." January 2020. https://www.buzzfeednews.com/article/annehelenpetersen/millennials-burnout-generation-debt-work

https://developingchild.harvard.edu/science/key-concepts/brain-architecture/

https://www.nice.org.uk/guidance/ng206 Published October 29th 2021

www.nicabm.com

http://vitaminsociety.org

https://www.youtube.com/watch?v=dLAi78hluFc Blue Eyed Brown Eyed Experiment

https://www.healthline.com/health/coercive-control Cali Este

https://www.nice.org.uk/news/article/nice-me-cfs-guideline-outlines-steps-for-better-diagnosis-and-management

https://www.ons.gov.uk/peoplepopulationandcommunity/crimeandjustice/bulletins/domesticabuseinenglandandwales/yearendingmarch2018#prevalence-of-domestic-abuse

Further Reading

You can access all research papers through Google Scholar:

John B. Arden, Lloyd Linford. (2009) *Brain Based Therapy with Adults*. Wiley.

Michael Argyle. (1994) *The Psychology of Interpersonal Behaviour*. Penguin.

Robert Dilts. (1990) *Beliefs; Pathways to Health and Well Being*. Portland USA. Metamorphous Press Pub.

Norman Doidge (2007) *The Brain Changes Itself*. New York. Viking Penguin.

Charles Duhigg. (2012) *The Power of Habit*. London. Random House.

Polly Evans. (2021) Improv Your Life. London. Hodder Studio

Susan Forward. (1986) Men Who Hate Women and The Women Who Love Them. NY USA. Bantam Press.

Daniel Goleman. (2003) *Destructive Emotions and how to overcome them. A dialogue with the Dalai Lama*. London. Bloomsbury.

Daniel Goleman. (1996) *Emotional Intelligence*. Great Britain. London. Bloomsbury.

David Goleman (2007) *Social Intelligence*. London. Arrow Books.

David Hamilton. (2015) *I Heart Me*. HayHouse.

Sandra Horley. (2000) *Power and Control: Why Charming Men Can Make Dangerous Lovers*. London. Vermilion.

Dr Michael Mosley. (2017) *The Clever Guts Diet*. Short Books Pub.

Sarah Myhill (2017) *"It's Mitochondria not Hypochondria"*. London. Hammersmith Health Books.

Steve Peters Dr. (2012) The Chimp Paradox. London. Vermillion.

Helen Petersen (2021) *Can't Even; How Millennials Became the Burnt Out Generation*. New York. Random House.

Stephen W Porges (2017) *The Pocket Guide to Polyvagal Theory*. New York. W.W. Norton.

V.S. Ramachandran. (2011) *The Tell Tale Brain*. London. Heinemann.

Dr. Megan Rossi (2021) *Eat More, Live Well: Enjoy Your Favourite Food and Boost Your Gut Health with The Diversity Diet*. Penguin Life.

Dr Megan Rossi. (2019) *Eat Yourself Healthy*. Penguin Life.

Francine Shapiro PhD. (2012) *Getting Past Your Past: EMDR Therapy*. New York. Rodale

Martin and Marion Shirran. (2012) *Pause Button Therapy*. Hay House.

Contacts

For an excellent coach contact: mark@markthecoach.co.uk

For an excellent RTT Therapist contact: www.catherinepaterson.co.uk

For EMDR to shift trauma, shock or recurring patterns, go to www. emdrassociation.org.uk

Jenna Green artist at www.jennagreenart.com

Alex Pink Media Production Expert www.pinkphotovideo.com

Alan Mead Coach/Trainer www.alanmead.co

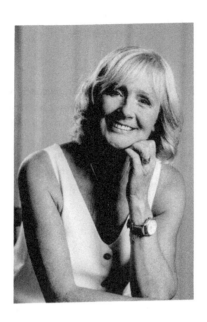

About the Author

Jan Rothney was subsequently diagnosed with ME in 2003, which came as a result of years of post-viral fatigue, other health conditions and living in an unhealthy environment. Jan recovered on her own, but a relapse in 2006 made her realise it wasn't enough to get physically better. She went on to run a clinic for ME and CFS / Post Viral Fatigue and has worked with up to a thousand clients to enable them to recover.

Now retired, Jan notes how fortunate she is to have such an array of amazing people in her life, including her husband, daughters, grandchildren and step children. She notes that she is deeply grateful every day that she has her health back and will never get ME / CFS again because she knows what to do to stop it.

Made in the USA
Las Vegas, NV
01 May 2024

89403656R00148